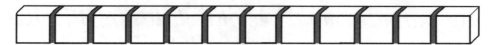

APhA's
Complete MATH Review for the

PHARMACY
TECHNICIAN

William A. Hopkins, Jr., Pharm.D., R.Ph., F.A.C.A.

President

Clinical Pharmacy Consultants of North Georgia

Big Canoe, Georgia

American Pharmaceutical Association
Washington, D.C.

APhA

To my loving parents, my awesome children Bill, Kim, Angie, and Abby and to my precious wife Patricia for her tireless love and dedication.

Notice

The author and the publisher have made a conscientious effort to ensure that the information in this book is accurate. However, the information should be used solely for course work, training in the pharmacy practice setting, and preparation for the national Pharmacy Technician Certification Examination. In no event should the information contained herein be used in connection with the actual services to be performed by pharmacy technicians.

This book is in no way authorized by or sponsored by the Pharmacy Technician Certification Board, Inc.

Acquiring Editor: Julian I. Graubart
Managing Editor: L. Luan Corrigan
Layout and Graphics: Kathryn A. Stromberger
Cover Designer: Mary Jane Hickey

© 2001 by the American Pharmaceutical Association
Published by the American Pharmaceutical Association
2215 Constitution Avenue, N.W.
Washington, DC 20037-2985
www.aphanet.org

To comment on this book via e-mail, send your message to the publisher at
aphabooks@mail.aphanet.org

How To Order This Book
By phone: 800-878-0729 (802-862-0095 from outside the United States)
VISA®, MasterCard®, and American Express® cards accepted.

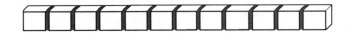

CONTENTS

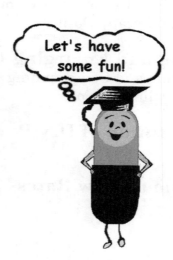

PREFACE

Have you ever said, **"I Can't Stand Math"?** For five decades, I have heard numerous pharmacists, technicians, nurses, and other healthcare practitioners make this statement. I have personally made similar comments. Unfortunately, most of my teachers were unable to make math interesting, practical, or fun. The aforementioned are reasons I finally decided to write a textbook that is easy to understand, practical, and entertaining.

By now, you have probably noticed I am writing to you personally and not in the "third person." It is important for me that you relax and know I recognize the barriers and fears you are experiencing in learning pharmacy calculations.

I will become your personal tutor and cheerleader throughout this publication and hopefully prove to you that math can be easy and enjoyable. More importantly, I want you to learn for life and not just for certification or for final examinations.

This textbook has been written in a self-instructional format so you can use it either while studying alone or in support of a formal course. It will also serve as a reference book throughout your pharmacy career.

When teaching math, I believe in the old acronym *K.I.S.S.,* which stands for "keep it simple, stupid." In sticking with this axiom, I promise to keep math at an uncomplicated level. In fact, you won't need to remember your algebra, geometry, trigonometry, or calculus to be successful with my techniques. Most problems in this book will be worked in the same manner using simple ratio and proportion.

In addition, I avoid formulas when teaching for several reasons. First, people tend to forget formulas or become confused when using them, leading to potential disasters. Second, many mistakes are made by people who are just plugging numbers into equations without understanding the logic behind the formulas. I want you to be totally confident your answer is correct when solving each and every problem.

We will start this book by performing the most basic math functions and slowly progressing to more challenging issues. It has been my experience that students who have difficulty with math frequently do not have a grasp of the fundamental concepts and then progress too quickly to the tougher questions.

With this in mind, ***please*** *master the basics and do not skip or hurry through early sections.* **Always** contact your instructor if you are having a problem with any concept, no matter how basic it may be. Each chapter will contain questions and examples that have nothing to do with pharmacy. The purpose of this is to help you relate what you are learning in this book to everyday life.

By so doing you will improve all of your math skills, not just those related to being a pharmacy technician. Finally, there will be a cumulative examination that will enable you to assess how far you have progressed. **Good luck** in your career in pharmacy and all other future endeavors. Now let's get started with a positive attitude about math and have a little fun.

William "Bill" A. Hopkins, Jr.
January 2001

I wish to thank the American Pharmaceutical Association for its leadership of our profession and for giving me the opportunity to write this textbook.

A special thanks to Dr. Loyd Allen, editor-in-chief of the International Journal of Pharmaceutical Compounding, *who has graciously permitted the use of innovative formulas from his publication. I am also grateful to the many pharmaceutical companies for the use of their package inserts and labels, and to the following technician educators for their review of the manuscript and helpful comments:*

Larry C. Nesmith, CPhT
Academy of Health Sciences
Fort Sam Houston
San Antonio, Texas

Douglas Scribner, CPhT
TVI Community College
Albuquerque, New Mexico

Karen R. Snipe, CPhT, MAEd
Trident Technical College
Charleston, South Carolina

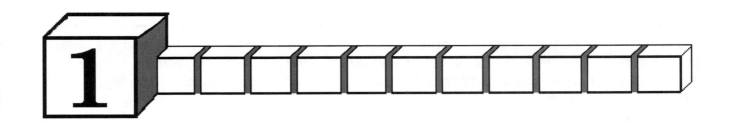

BACK TO BASICS

*W*elcome to the second step in learning pharmaceutical calculations. The first step was reading the Preface, which you probably skipped if you are like most of my students! I will wait a few minutes while you go back and read those very important pages.

Now that you have mastered Step One, let's start learning the important fundamentals of math necessary for future chapters and for your work in pharmacy.

OBJECTIVES

Upon mastery of Chapter 1 you will be able to:

Express Arabic numbers as Roman numerals.
Express Roman numerals as Arabic numbers.
Add, subtract, multiply, and divide common fractions.
Add, subtract, multiply, and divide decimal fractions.
Convert common fractions to decimal fractions.
Convert decimal fractions to common fractions.

Arabic and Roman Numerals

All of you are familiar with the "Arabic" system of notation, the basic ten figures, 0,1,2,3,4,5,6,7,8,9. These figures are arranged in various orders with different values assigned to the digits according to the location they occupy in a row. An example would be the numbers 21 and 210. You all know from your first grade education that the "2" in 21 has a value of 20, but in 210 the "2" stands for 200.

HERE COME
THE ROMANS!!!

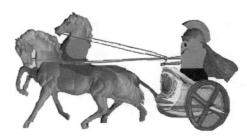

There is another system of notation known as "Roman numerals" that is a lot older than I am! This system dates back thousands of years and is still being used by some practitioners today. You are probably asking yourself "why" this is occurring. The primary reason is because of an ancient system of measurement known as the "apothecaries'."

This method requires the use of Roman numerals. An example would be writing the abbreviation of 6 grains which is written as gr.vi. The apothecaries' system is discouraged in contemporary pharmacy practice, but you need to understand Roman numerals because they still appear on many prescriptions and compounding formulas.

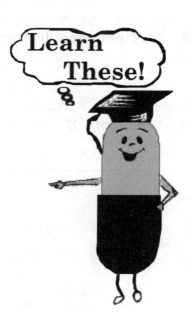

The Roman system utilizes eight letters to designate numbers. (Throughout this book, my assistant, Wily Willie, will point out important things for you.) Before you continue, take a little time and memorize these Roman numerals and their Arabic equivalents:

$$\frac{1}{2} = \text{ss}$$
$$1 = \text{I} \quad \text{or} \quad \text{i}$$
$$5 = \text{V} \quad \text{or} \quad \text{v}$$
$$10 = \text{X} \quad \text{or} \quad \text{x}$$
$$50 = \text{L} \quad \text{or} \quad \text{l}$$
$$100 = \text{C} \quad \text{or} \quad \text{c}$$
$$500 = \text{D} \quad \text{or} \quad \text{d}$$
$$1000 = \text{M} \quad \text{or} \quad \text{m}$$

Now that you have mastered Roman equivalents, it is time to create Arabic numbers from Roman numerals and vice versa. Unfortunately, I have bad news for you because the two systems are very different in how they work.

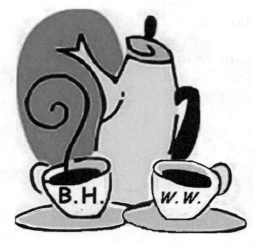

For example, the number 40 cannot be written as XXXX, nor can the number 15 be written as VVV.

Why?

Because there are eight rules of Roman numerals you have to learn before we continue.

So get to work and memorize the rules on the next page while Wily Willie and I take a break.

Roman Numeral Rules

1. When a letter is repeated, its value is repeated.

   II = 1 + 1 = 2 and XXX = 10 + 10 + 10 = 30

   So, you ask,"why isn't XXXX equal to 40?"

   Keep reading, you will figure it out.

   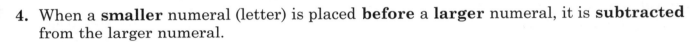

2. A letter cannot be repeated more than three times.

   So XXXX is not equal to 40 and VVVVv is not equal to 25. But what about VVV?

3. V, L, and D are never repeated.

   This explains why VVV is not equal to 15, nor is VV equal to 10.

4. When a **smaller** numeral (letter) is placed **before** a **larger** numeral, it is **subtracted** from the larger numeral.

   IV = 4   IX = 9   XL = 40   CD = 400   CM = 900

5. When a **smaller** numeral is placed **after** a larger numeral, it is **added** to the larger numeral.

   VI = 6   XI = 11   LX = 60   MC = 1100   MD = 1500

6. V, L, and D are never subtracted from larger numbers.

   So VL is not equal to 45 and LM is not equal to 950.

7. Never subtract more than one numeral.

   So IIX is not equal to 8 and XXXC is not equal to 70.

8. Use I before V and X (only the next two highest numerals). The same is true for X and C (i.e., X before L and C; C before D and M).

   IV = 4 and IX = 9 **but** IC is **not** equal to 99

   XC = 90 **but** XM is **not** equal to 990

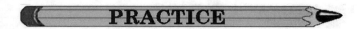

PRACTICE

*Please work all problems in this book with a **pencil** so corrections can be easily made.*

1. Write the corresponding Arabic or Roman numbers for the following:

(a)	CC	=	(e)	XL	=	(i)	XII	=
(b)	LL	=	(f)	VD	=	(j)	IIC	=
(c)	MMM	=	(g)	LV	=			
(d)	CCCC	=	(h)	IM	=			

If you had trouble with a–j, restudy rules 1–8 before continuing.

(k)	XXII	=	(q)	DXV	=	(w)	47	=
(l)	LI	=	(r)	XXIX	=	(x)	62	=
(m)	CX	=	(s)	CDXLV	=	(y)	480	=
(n)	CL	=	(t)	XIVI	=	(z)	1999	=
(o)	LXVI	=	(u)	18	=			
(p)	MIV	=	(v)	34	=			

▼▼▼▼▼ *The answers to all problems can be found in the answer key starting on page 160.* ▼▼▼▼▼

Fractions

*A fraction indicates a portion of a whole number. There are two types of fractions discussed in this chapter. They are the **common** fractions and the **decimal** fractions. Let's first look at common fractions.*

Common Fractions

A common fraction is an expression of division with one number placed over another. Examples of common fractions are $\frac{1}{2}$ and $\frac{3}{4}$.

*The bottom number is referred to as the **denominator** and the top number is the **numerator**. In these examples, the numerators are the numbers 1 and 3 and the denominators are the numbers 2 and 4. The denominator represents the total number of parts that the whole number is divided into. In the example $\frac{1}{2}$, the whole number is divided into 2 parts. In the example $\frac{3}{4}$, the whole number is divided into 4 parts. The numerator tells us how many of those parts we are concerned with.*

Are you confused?

Let's take the first example $\frac{1}{2}$, and discuss it. All of you know what $\frac{1}{2}$ means. If I said you have $\frac{1}{2}$ dollar, you know you have 50 cents. You knew that from everyday experiences. Even though you knew the answer, did you really understand the total concept? It is important to have a thorough comprehension of how fractions work before we get to Chapter 3 and start learning ratio and proportion. So take a few minutes and think about the definition of a common fraction and how it relates to the dollar example.

If the denominator of $\frac{1}{2}$ is 2, this means that the total number is divided into 2 parts. In the case of a dollar, the 100 cents are divided into 2 parts, each containing 50 cents. The numerator tells us how many of those parts we are concerned with. So with a numerator of 1, we will have 1 of the 2 parts each containing 50 cents.

How many cents would be in $\frac{3}{4}$ of a dollar? Think about this based on our discussion, not on what is in your "memory bank." The denominator is 4, meaning the 100 cents in a dollar are broken into 4 parts each containing 25 cents. The numerator is 3, which means you are concerned with 3 parts or a total of 75 cents (i.e., 3 x 25 = 75).

Now that you think this is so easy, why don't you try one?
Question: How many cents would be in $\frac{13}{20}$ of a dollar?
(OK, OK, I had the easy ones, but see if you can solve this in the space below before looking at the solution.)

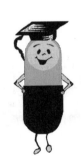

Solution: 1 dollar is equal to 100 cents. 100 cents divided by 20 (the denominator) equals 5 cents per part. Multiply 5 cents per part by 13 (i.e., the numerator) and the answer is **65 cents.**

Types of Common Fractions

In the previous section, we were discussing common fractions in a form sometimes referred to as **proper** *fractions. These are fractions where the numerator is smaller than the denominator, that is, $\frac{1}{2}$, $\frac{3}{4}$, etc. There are several other types of fractions you need to know for future reference.*

Improper fractions *are fractions where the numerator is larger than the denominator.*
Examples: $\frac{9}{7}$ $\frac{13}{12}$ $\frac{37}{18}$

Improper fractions are frequently used when adding, subtracting, multiplying, and dividing with fractions.

Mixed fractions *are combinations of whole numbers and proper fractions.*

Examples: $1\frac{1}{2}$ and $3\frac{3}{4}$

Mixed fractions must be converted to improper fractions before calculating.

Calculating with Fractions

Before calculating with fractions, make sure all mixed fractions are changed to improper fractions. This is easily done by simply multiplying the whole number times the denominator and then adding the numerator and placing the resulting number over the denominator.

Example: $4\frac{1}{2}$ —multiply the whole number (4) times the denominator (2), which equals 8. Now add the numerator (1) to give the number 9. Simply place the 9 over the original denominator (2) and your answer is $\frac{9}{2}$. So, $4\frac{1}{2}$ is equal to $\frac{9}{2}$.

Now you need to try one.

Question: Convert this mixed fraction to an improper fraction: $12\frac{5}{8}$ = ?

Solution: Multiply 12 times the denominator (8) = 96
Add 96 to the numerator (5) = 101
Place the 101 over the original denominator (8)
And the answer is $12\frac{5}{8}$ = $\frac{101}{8}$

Multiplying Fractions

*I am starting with **multiplication** because it is the easiest process of all. To multiply fractions, be sure to convert all whole numbers to improper fractions.*

Example: 5 = $\frac{5}{1}$

Make sure all mixed fractions are converted to improper fractions.

Example: $2\frac{1}{2}$ = $\frac{5}{2}$

Now all you have to do is multiply the numerators times each other, and do the same for the denominators. Let's use these examples to multiply 5 times $2\frac{1}{2}$.

Solution: 5 × $2\frac{1}{2}$ = **?** *(Convert these to improper fractions.)*

$\frac{5}{1}$ × $\frac{5}{2}$ = $\frac{25}{2}$ *(Multiply numerators and denominators.)*

The answer $\frac{25}{2}$ is correct, but the proper way of reporting this answer is in the form of a mixed fraction, or $12\frac{1}{2}$. To calculate the mixed fraction, simply divide the numerator (25) by the denominator (2), which gives you 12 with a remainder of 1. Make sure you put the remainder (1) over the denominator (2).

Tag, it's your turn to try one! Multiply $5\frac{7}{8}$ times $\frac{3}{5}$.

Solution:

$$5\frac{7}{8} \quad \times \quad \frac{3}{5} \quad = \quad ?$$

$$\frac{47}{8} \quad \times \quad \frac{3}{5} \quad = \quad ?$$

$$\frac{47}{8} \quad \times \quad \frac{3}{5} \quad = \quad \frac{141}{40} \quad = \quad 3\frac{21}{40}$$

Now why don't we try to put these fractions into a real-world problem.

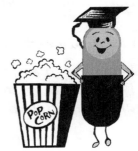

Example: Yesterday I bought a box of 6 microwave popcorn packets.
I noticed that each packet weighed $6\frac{3}{4}$ ounces.
How much did the entire box weigh?

Solution:

$$6\frac{3}{4} \quad \times \quad 6 \quad = \quad ?$$

$$\frac{27}{4} \quad \times \quad \frac{6}{1} \quad = \quad \frac{162}{4} \quad = \quad 40\frac{2}{4} \text{ ounces}$$

Whenever possible, try to reduce fractions to the lowest terms. In this example, the answer $40\frac{2}{4}$ is correct, but the more cosmetically correct answer is $40\frac{1}{2}$. To reduce the fraction $\frac{2}{4}$ to lowest terms, divide the numerator and denominator by the highest number that will divide into each number an even number of times. In this case, the best number is 2. $\frac{2 \div 2}{4 \div 2} = \frac{1}{2}$ **Your final answer will become $40\frac{1}{2}$ ounces.**

Dividing Fractions

Dividing fractions is almost as easy as multiplying, but there is one big difference. When you divide fractions, you will do everything just like you are multiplying until you get to the last step. Before you multiply the numerators and denominators, you need to invert the divisor (the number you're going to divide by). Let's look at an example.

$$\frac{7}{12} \div 5 = ?$$

$$\frac{7}{12} \div \frac{5}{1} = ?$$

As you can see, the process so far is the same. Now for the big difference. In division, you invert the divisor before multiplying. I like to change the sign from ($\div$) to ($\times$) when I invert the divisor. This is how it looks:

$$\frac{7}{12} \times \frac{1}{5} = \frac{7}{60}$$

At this point I want to stress with you what I think is the most important math skill you can learn. The skill is called **estimating**. Frequently, errors can be avoided if practitioners simply estimate correct answers. In this example, we were dividing a number with a value less than 1 by 5. It is easy to predict that the answer will be a small number (i.e., less than 1). If you were to make a math error and not invert the divisor in this problem, **your answer would be almost 3.**

It's time again for you to show me how smart you are!

Question: Now I just bought a 20-ounce box of Cheerios®. How many meals can I eat out of this box if I eat $3\frac{1}{3}$ ounces of Cheerios every morning for breakfast? (Write your answer below before looking at the solution.)

Solution: *Did you* **estimate** *your answer before working this problem? If not, you are hopeless.* *Just kidding!*

Learning to estimate is hard to do, but take my word it is well worth the effort. I estimated by saying I have 20 ounces divided by about 3, so the correct answer is approximately 6 or 7 (plus or minus a few Cheerios).

$$20 \div 3\tfrac{1}{3} = ?$$

$$\tfrac{20}{1} \div \tfrac{10}{3} = ?$$

$$\tfrac{20}{1} \times \tfrac{3}{10} = \tfrac{60}{10} = \tfrac{6}{1} = \quad \text{6 servings of Cheerios}$$

Adding and Subtracting Fractions

Adding and subtracting fractions requires more work than multiplying and dividing. When adding and subtracting, you must find a common denominator for every fraction. This process must be done before you can proceed with calculating the answer. In solving for a **common denominator**, *remember the fraction will be exactly the same if you multiply or divide the numerator and denominator by the same number.*

Example: Multiply the numerator and denominator in the fraction $\frac{1}{2}$ by 5. Your answer is $\frac{5}{10}$. You all know that $\frac{5}{10}$ is the same as $\frac{1}{2}$, so the fractions are equal. If you took the fraction $\frac{7}{21}$ and divided the numerator and denominator by 7, you will have the fraction $\frac{1}{3}$. This means that $\frac{7}{21}$ and $\frac{1}{3}$ are equal fractions. Now let's solve for **common denominators** and start adding and subtracting fractions.

Question: Add the following fractions: $\frac{5}{8} + \frac{1}{6} + \frac{2}{3} = ?$

Think about the steps involved and then look at the next page.

Step 1. Make sure all numbers are proper or improper fractions (no mixed fractions).

Step 2. Find common denominators for all fractions. Simply take multiples of the "largest" of the 3 denominators until you come up with a number that all denominators will divide into an *even* number of times. In this example, the largest denominator is 8. Multiples of 8 are: 16, 24, 32, 40, 48, 56, etc.

Which of these numbers is the lowest number that all 3 denominators will divide into an even number of times?

The answer is 24.

This means 24 is our lowest common denominator (LCD). The number 48 would also be OK, but higher numbers create more work and greater chances of making errors.

Step 3. Create new fractions with all having the same common denominator. Remember earlier I told you the "value" of fractions does not change if you multiply or divide both the numerator and denominator by the "same" number.

Now let's change all the fractions so they all have denominators of 24.

$\frac{5}{8} = \frac{?}{24}$ (The new denominator 24 is 3 times larger than the 8 in $\frac{5}{8}$. If the new denominator is 3 times larger, then you need to also multiply the numerator by 3 to have equal fractions. So $\frac{5}{8}$ equals $\frac{15}{24}$.)

Now you solve for $\frac{1}{6}$ and $\frac{2}{3}$.

Solution: $\qquad \frac{1}{6} = \frac{?}{24}$

$\qquad\qquad \frac{1}{6} = \frac{4}{24}$

Solution: $\qquad \frac{2}{3} = \frac{?}{24}$

$\qquad\qquad \frac{2}{3} = \frac{16}{24}$

Step 4. Add or subtract the numerators and place them over the common denominator.

DO NOT add the denominators.

$$\frac{15}{24} + \frac{4}{24} + \frac{16}{24} = \frac{?}{24} = \frac{35}{24}$$

Step 5. Reduce answer to lowest terms or to a mixed fraction.

$$\frac{35}{24} = 1\frac{11}{24}$$

It's show time! Try to solve this one.

Question: My Uncle Dudley is a farmer. Last year he sold his corn crop to 3 different merchants. One merchant bought $\frac{3}{16}$ of Uncle Dudley's crop, another bought $\frac{1}{8}$, and the third merchant bought $\frac{13}{24}$ of the crop. How much of the total crop did they buy?

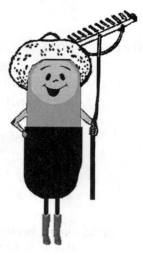

Solution: **Step 1.** All numbers are proper fractions.

Step 2. The common denominator is a multiple of 24 and is 48.

Step 3. Create new fractions with a denominator of 48:

$$\frac{3}{16} = \frac{9}{48}$$

$$\frac{13}{24} = \frac{26}{48}$$

$$\frac{1}{8} = \frac{6}{48}$$

Step 4. Add the numerators and place them over the common denominator:

$$\frac{9}{48} + \frac{26}{48} + \frac{6}{48} = \frac{?}{48} = \frac{41}{48}$$

Step 5. Already reduced to lowest terms.

Question: Now that you think you have mastered this process, why don't you tell me how much of Uncle Dudley's crop was left over after the merchants took their $\frac{41}{48}$.

Solution: **Step 1.** The total crop would be equal to all the parts (i.e., $\frac{48}{48}$, which is 1).

Step 2. The common denominator is 48.

Step 3. Both fractions $\frac{41}{48}$ and $\frac{48}{48}$ have the same denominator.

Step 4. Subtract numerators $\frac{48}{48} - \frac{41}{48} = \frac{?}{48} = \frac{7}{48}$

Step 5. Already reduced to lowest terms. My uncle had $\frac{7}{48}$ of his crop left.

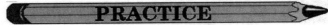

PRACTICE

2. Multiply and reduce answers to lowest terms.

(a) $7 \times \frac{1}{12} = $ **?** (d) $\frac{1}{500} \times 5 = $ **?**

(b) $\frac{3}{5} \times \frac{1}{5} = $ **?** (e) $8\frac{3}{4} \times \frac{3}{120} = $ **?**

(c) $1\frac{1}{6} \times 2\frac{1}{2} = $ **?**

3. Divide and reduce answers to lowest terms.

(a) $\frac{3}{5} \div \frac{4}{5} = $ **?** (d) $11 \div 3\frac{3}{4} = $ **?**

(b) $19\frac{1}{4} \div 3 = $ **?** (e) $\frac{1}{8} \div 8 = $ **?**

(c) $\frac{1}{50} \div \frac{1}{200} = $ **?**

4. Add and reduce to lowest terms.

(a) $\frac{3}{8} + \frac{5}{16} = $ **?**

(b) $\frac{9}{13} + \frac{1}{3} = $ **?**

(c) $1\frac{5}{8} + 3\frac{3}{4} + 5\frac{3}{10} = $ **?**

(d) $10\frac{1}{2} + 5 + 6\frac{1}{3} = $ **?**

(e) $3\frac{2}{3} + 5\frac{1}{2} + \frac{5}{11} = $ **?**

5. Subtract and reduce to lowest terms.

(a) $\frac{4}{5} - \frac{3}{10} = $ **?** (d) $\frac{3}{100} - \frac{1}{150} = $ **?**

(b) $5\frac{1}{12} - \frac{2}{3} = $ **?** (e) $7\frac{2}{5} - \frac{2}{3} = $ **?**

(c) $11\frac{3}{4} - 9\frac{1}{2} = $ **?**

6. During the past few weeks I have purchased bananas on four different occasions. The weights were $\frac{3}{4}$ pound, $\frac{1}{2}$ pound, 2 pounds, and $1\frac{5}{8}$ pounds. How many pounds of bananas did I buy?

7. From your answer in Question 6, how many pounds of bananas have I consumed if I still have $1\frac{1}{2}$ pounds of uneaten bananas?

OK, OK, so you're getting tired of bananas and Cheerios! Let's try a few of these problems and relate them to your career in pharmacy. Please note that the math is the same. We will only change the units to pharmaceutical and medical terms.

8. A pharmacist buys sulfur powder at different times in quantities of $\frac{3}{8}$ pound, $1\frac{1}{2}$ pounds, $\frac{3}{16}$ pound, and 2 pounds. How much sulfur did she buy?

9. Using your answer from Question 8, how much sulfur would remain if the pharmacy technician compounded three prescriptions of mange powder, each containing $1\frac{1}{4}$ pounds of sulfur?

10. A bottle of children's cough syrup contains 24 teaspoons of medication. If the dose of the syrup for a 6-year-old is $\frac{3}{4}$ teaspoon, how many doses are in the bottle?

11. A cardiac patient taking $\frac{1}{150}$ grain nitroglycerin tablets took two tablets in the morning, one in the afternoon, and two in the evening. How many grains of nitroglycerin did the patient receive?

12. A prescription for 30 capsules requires a total of $\frac{3}{16}$ ounce of a potent narcotic. How much of the narcotic would be contained in each capsule?

▼▼▼▼▼ *The answers to all problems can be found in the answer key starting on page 160.* ▼▼▼▼▼

Decimal Fractions

Decimals are fractions with a denominator of any multiple of 10 (e.g., 10, 100, 1000, 10,000). Decimal fractions differ from the common fractions we previously discussed in that decimal fractions signify the denominator with a decimal point placed to the left of the numerator. This probably doesn't make a whole lot of sense, so let me give you several examples.

Example: $\frac{9}{10}$ written as a decimal fraction is 0.9

The first place to the right of the decimal signifies tenths, the next place signifies hundredths, the next thousandths, then ten thousandths, etc. Always place a zero to the left of the decimal point if there is not a whole number occupying that position.
Examples: 0.35 and 0.00487. The example $\frac{9}{10}$ is written 0.9 and is read "nine-tenths." In the case of a mixed fraction like $3\frac{1}{100}$, you would write it as 3.01 and read it as "three and one-hundredth."

Example: $\frac{125}{1000}$ written as a decimal fraction is 0.125

Would a zero to the right of 0.125 change the value of this decimal? The answer is *NO* because 0.1250 would be $\frac{1250}{10000}$ so when it is reduced it becomes $\frac{125}{1000}$.

Would a zero to the left of the 1 in 0.125 change the value of the decimal? The answer is *absolutely YES* because 0.0125 is $\frac{125}{10000}$ and can't be reduced to $\frac{125}{1000}$.

Question: Which of the following is the largest number: 0.12 or 0.0978?

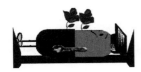

You might have selected 0.0978 and you might also have killed the patient!
The number 0.12 is also written $\frac{12}{100}$. The decimal 0.0978 is equal to $\frac{978}{10000}$. So far it might be hard to tell which is larger because these two fractions are very different in appearance.

Gee, I wonder if there is a way to make the fractions look similar. What if we made $\frac{12}{100}$ and $\frac{978}{10000}$ have common denominators?

The common denominator would be 10,000. Thus $\frac{12}{100}$ would become $\frac{1200}{10000}$ which is larger than $\frac{978}{10000}$. This means 0.12 is larger than 0.0978.

CONVERTING COMMON FRACTIONS TO DECIMALS

To convert fractions to decimals, divide the numerator by the denominator.

Question: If you have the fraction $\frac{1}{2}$, how do you convert it to a decimal fraction?

**All right, I know you can do this with a calculator,
but to better understand the process, please work it below.**

Solution: Take the numerator (1) and divide it by the denominator (2).
Your answer is 0.5 or $\frac{5}{10}$, read *five-tenths*.

Question: Now that you think you have mastered the process, please show me the
decimal fraction value for $\frac{3}{8}$.

Solution: Divide the numerator (3) by the denominator (8), which will give you
the decimal fraction 0.375; this is equal to $\frac{375}{1000}$ and is read
three hundred and seventy-five thousandths.

Question: **Let's try a tougher one.** Write the decimal fraction for $132\frac{3}{4}$.

Solution: Divide 3 by 4 which gives you the decimal 0.75, and then place the whole
number 132 to the left of the decimal point. Our new decimal fraction is
132.75 and is read *one hundred and thirty-two and seventy-five hundreths*.

CONVERTING DECIMALS TO COMMON FRACTIONS

***To convert decimals to common fractions, simply express the decimal as a fraction
and reduce it to the lowest terms.***

Question: Convert 0.25 to a common fraction.

Solution: 0.25 is the same as $\frac{25}{100}$. Reduce this number to the lowest terms, and you
will have the common fraction $\frac{1}{4}$.

To check your answer of $\frac{1}{4}$, divide 1 by 4 and you will have the decimal fraction 0.25.

Question: Convert 0.125 to a common fraction.

Solution: 0.125 expressed as a common fraction is $\frac{125}{1000}$ and can be reduced to $\frac{1}{8}$. Check your answer by dividing 1 by 8.

Question: Express 111.004 as a common fraction.

Solution: 0.004 expressed as a common fraction is $\frac{4}{1000}$ and can be reduced to $\frac{1}{250}$. The reduced common fraction is $111\frac{1}{250}$.

ADDING AND SUBTRACTING DECIMAL FRACTIONS

When adding and subtracting decimal fractions, make sure the decimal points line up vertically. Add additional zeros to the right and left of the numbers to make all numbers of equal length and to avoid errors.

Example: 0.135 + 1.21 + 153.1 = ?

Solution:

```
    000.135
    001.210
  + 153.100
    154.445
```

Question: Solve the following: 14.012 − 3.11 = ?

Solution:
```
    14.012
  − 03.110
answer 10.902
```

MULTIPLYING DECIMAL FRACTIONS

Count the total number of decimal places in the numbers multiplied and place the decimal point in the product (answer) to the left of the total number of places counted (count from the right).

CONFUSED? Let's look at an example to better explain this procedure.

Example: Solve the following: $216.3 \times 8.25 = ?$

$$
\begin{array}{r}
216.3 \quad \text{(1 decimal place)} \\
\times \quad \underline{8.25} \quad \text{(2 decimal places)} \\
1784475
\end{array}
$$

Why is this answer incorrect?

Answer: Because the decimal point has not been correctly placed.

The correct answer is 1,784.475 because there was a total of three decimal places in the two numbers multiplied and it is necessary to place the decimal in the answer 3 places starting from the right.

DIVIDING DECIMAL FRACTIONS

When dividing decimals, move the decimal places in the divisor and the dividend to the right to create "whole" numbers. Make sure you move each decimal an EQUAL number of places and add zeros if necessary.

Example: $3.5 \div 1.5 = ?$
$35 \div 15 = 2.333333$ (round off to 2 decimal places) $= 2.33$

Here, both decimals were moved 1 place to the right, but what would you do with the following example?

Example: $6.85 \div 4.6 = ?$
$685 \div 460 = 1.48913$ (round off to 2 decimal places) $= 1.49$

Since the decimal in 6.85 was moved 2 places to the right it was necessary to add an extra zero to 4.6 so the decimal could also be moved an equal number of places.

Have you noticed I do not put a decimal point to the right of whole numbers? This is appropriate because there is no need to place it there.

Question: Please divide the following numbers and round off your answer.
$22.87 \div 0.107 = ?$

Solution: $22.87 \div 0.107 = ?$
$22870 \div 107 = 213.73831 = 213.74 = 214$

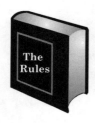

I have my own rule for rounding off numbers that will keep your answers within approximately 1% of the correct answer. In the first two examples I rounded off two decimal places. I do this whenever there is one whole number to the left of the decimal place. If you have two whole numbers, then round off to one decimal place and in the last question, we had three whole numbers, so I dropped all the decimal places.

There are some areas of pharmacy practice (though rare) that may require you to be more accurate.

MULTIPLYING AND DIVIDING DECIMALS BY POWERS OF TEN

When multiplying decimals by powers of ten, move the decimal point as many places to the RIGHT as there are zeros in the multiplier. When dividing by powers of ten, move the decimal point to the LEFT as many places as there are zeros in the divisor.

Examples: $4.83 \times 10 = ?$ (move decimal one place to the right) = 48.3

$0.035 \times 1000 = ?$ (move decimal three places to the right) = 35

This is especially good for estimating your answers. Example: $2.1 \times 300 = ?$
In this example, move the decimal point 2 places to the right and multiply by three
(i.e., $2.1 \times 300 = 210 \times 3 = 630$). This takes some practice, but it is a great skill
to master and is worth the extra effort.

Examples: $72.62 \div 10 = ?$ (move the decimal one place to the left) $= 7.262$

$367.3 \div 100 = ?$ (move the decimal two places to the left) $= 3.673$

Question: I bought a 5.5-pound roast and you laughed and said you had a bull that weighed 4000 times that amount. Estimate the weight of the animal—is there a possibility you might be exaggerating?

Solution: $5.5 \times 4000 = ?$ (Because there are three zeros, move the decimal three places to the right and multiply by four), that is,
$5500 \times 4 = 22,000$ pounds

**I think you were "shooting the bull"!
(no pun intended)**

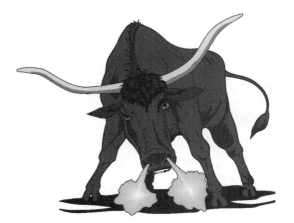

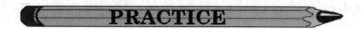

PRACTICE

13. Add the following decimal fractions:

(a)   15   +   1.5   +   0.15   +   150   =   ?

(b)   3.25   +   13.091   +   0.18   =   ?

(c)   0.38   +   0.097   +   0.0062   =   ?

(d)   22.0008 +   8.022   =   ?

14. Subtract the following decimal fractions:

(a) 32   −   1.0009   =   ?   (c)   491.08   −   321.008   =   ?

(b) 2.52   −   0.333   =   ?   (d)   0.0678   −   0.00678   =   ?

15. Divide the following decimal fractions:

(a) 23.8   ÷   0.294   =   ?   (c)   341.44   ÷   0.37   =   ?

(b) 0.91   ÷   8.27   =   ?   (d)   68.2   ÷   2000   =   ?
                                         (try to guess this one before working it)

16. Multiply the following decimal fractions:

(a) 0.003 ×   0.09   =   ?   (c)   100.25   ×   100.35   =   ?

(b) 54.5 ×   25.12   =   ?   (d)   1336   ×   10,000   =   ?
                                         (try to guess this one before working it)

I have an idea. Why don't we put the entire chapter together and create some stress, I mean some confidence!

 Tip   Make sure all numbers are in one system before calculating.

17. Solve the following and reduce to lowest terms:

(a)   XXIV   ×   3.25   =   ?

(b)   26.23   × $6\frac{7}{12}$ =   ?

(c)   LXVI   +   41.9   + $333\frac{1}{2}$ =   ?

(d)   cxiiiss   times $8\frac{3}{8}$ =   ?

(e)   LXVII   –   XLII   =   ?   (give answer in Roman numerals)

(f)   17.1   ÷ $4\frac{3}{8}$ =   ?

(g) $3\frac{3}{4}$ ÷   3.089   =   ?

(h)   5.029   × $19\frac{7}{8}$ =   ?

18. A bottle of olive oil contains 96 teaspoons of oil. If you average putting $4\frac{4}{5}$ teaspoons of olive oil on a salad, how many salads can you prepare?

19. If you prepare $8\frac{1}{2}$ meals from a box of oatmeal that weighs XXXII ounces, how many ounces of oatmeal would be in each meal (express as a decimal fraction)?

20. If the average pharmacy technician can prepare CIX prescriptions per day, how many technicians would be required to prepare MDCXXXV prescriptions?

21. A pharmacy technician has 100 grams of drug A on hand. How much will remain if she fills three prescriptions for capsules containing the following:

        Rx 1   #30 capsules each containing $1\frac{1}{4}$ grams of drug A

        Rx 2   #15 capsules each containing 2.75 grams of drug A

        Rx 3   #10 capsules each containing iss grams of drug A

22. How many capsules containing $1\frac{3}{4}$ grams of drug A can be prepared from the remainder of drug A in Question 21 (give answer as a decimal fraction)?

23. If a combination cold capsule contains 32.5 milligrams of drug B, $15\frac{3}{8}$ milligrams of drug C, 75.5 milligrams of drug D, and $118\frac{1}{8}$ milligrams of drug E, how many total milligrams (expressed in Roman numerals) would be contained in each capsule?

24. How many 0.00055-gram doses can be made from $\frac{3}{4}$ gram of a drug?

25. If 1 kilogram of antiseptic powder costs $350, how much will 0.001 kilogram cost?

▼▼▼▼▼ *The answers to all problems can be found in the answer key starting on page 160.* ▼▼▼▼▼

NOW, IF YOU UNDERSTAND CHAPTER 1 REAL WELL,
   LET'S GO FIGURE OUT WHAT THESE GRAMS, MILLIGRAMS,
KILOGRAMS, AND CHEERIOS® ARE ALL ABOUT.

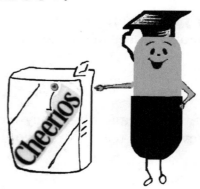

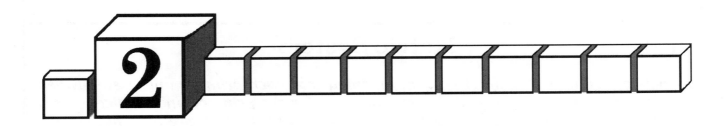

SYSTEMS OF MEASUREMENT

In Chapter 1, we reviewed the fundamentals of mathematics that will be used throughout this textbook. Before we get into the "meat and potatoes" of pharmaceutical calculations, I want you to master one more foundation area: the systems of measurement.

Most textbooks focus on the three systems of measurement (metric, apothecary, and avoirdupois), but I will focus on the "metric" and briefly mention the other two systems. My reasoning is that the metric system has been adopted and mandated in the United States and throughout the world as the standard for pharmaceutical and medical calculations.

In addition, the U.S. Pharmacopeial Convention, the National Association of Boards of Pharmacy, and other "standard setting" organizations have embraced the metric system as the sole system of measurement. As a pharmacy technician, you need to master the metric system, but you should also know there are other systems just in case they appear on a prescription or an old compounding formula.

OBJECTIVES

Upon mastery of Chapter 2 you will be able to:

Understand the guidelines for metric notation.
Recognize the apothecary and avoirdupois systems of measurement.
Perform basic math functions using the systems of measurement.
Relate the metric system to "household" equivalents utilized by patients.

---

*T*he metric system has three primary units:

- ❑ the **meter,** *which measures length,*

- ❑ the **liter,** *which is used for volume, and*

- ❑ the **gram,** *which measures weight.*

Metric System

The metric system is a decimal system, meaning that each primary unit is subdivided by multiples of ten. In the metric system, prefixes for the primary units indicate what segment of the unit is being considered. There are more than 16 prefixes, but since I can't remember most of them, and more importantly you will rarely use the majority of them, I will only focus on the following four:

S o Here Are

The Important Ones !!!

kilo = 1000 or one thousand

centi = $\frac{1}{100}$ or 0.01 or one hundredth

milli = $\frac{1}{1000}$ or 0.001 or one thousandth

micro = $\frac{1}{1000000}$ or 0.000001 or one millionth

So how do all these prefixes and primary units relate to pharmacy?

Here are metric measurements and abbreviations you will encounter frequently in everyday medical and pharmacy practice:

LENGTH

meter   (m)

centimeter   (cm) $\frac{1}{100}$ of a meter

millimeter   (mm) $\frac{1}{1000}$ of a meter

WEIGHT

gram   (g or Gm)

milligram   (mg) $\frac{1}{1000}$ of a gram

microgram (mcg *or* μg) $\frac{1}{1000000}$ of a gram

kilogram   (kg *or* Kg)   1,000 grams

VOLUME

liter   (l or L)

milliliter   (ml or mL) $\frac{1}{1000}$ of a liter

A cubic centimeter (cc) is sometimes used by practitioners to denote a milliliter.

Guidelines for Metric Notation

1. **Always place the number before the abbreviation.**
   8 ml not ml 8

2. **Place a zero to the left of the decimal when the decimal fraction is less than 1.**
   Digoxin 0.125 mg not digoxin .125 mg. (The zero draws attention to the decimal and decreases the possibility of giving the wrong dose; in this case, 125 mg might be given if the decimal is not noticed.)

3. **Never place a zero to the right of the decimal place** when you have a whole number.
   A patient weighs 11 kg not 11.0 kg. (The zero in this example may mask the decimal, and the weight may be read as 110 kg.)

4. **Always use decimals to reflect fractions when using the metric system.**
   3.5 mg not $3\frac{1}{2}$ mg.

5. **Avoid unnecessary zeros.**
   60.02000 g should be written 60.02 g because the last 3 zeros have no value, but zeros between whole numbers are very important to accurately interpret the numbers.

6. **Always think carefully when converting from subunits.** When going from a small unit to a larger unit, make sure your number *decreases* proportionately.
   Convert 5,675 mg to grams.
   A gram is 1,000 times larger than a milligram, so the number to the left of the primary unit must be divided by 1,000. In this example, 5,675 mg = 5.675 g.

7. **When converting from a large unit to a smaller unit,** make sure your number *increases* proportionately.
   Convert 72 kg to grams.
   A gram is 1,000 times smaller than a kg, so the number to the left of the primary unit (i.e., gram) must be multiplied by 1,000.
   In this example, 72 kg = 72,000 g.

8. **When multiplying metric values by multiples of ten,** move the decimal point one place to the *right* for each zero in the multiplier.
   10   ×   84.67   =   846.7
   1000 ×   0.325   =   325

9. **When dividing metric values by multiples of ten,** move the decimal point one place to the *left* for each zero in the divisor.
   74.67 ÷   100   =   0.7467
   0.67 ÷ 1,000   =   0.00067

10. **When in doubt, check it out!** Always check when clarification is needed. A one decimal error in dosing can frequently be **fatal** to a patient, so be careful.

▼▼▼▼▼

PRACTICE

1. Convert the following metric units:

   (a)   25 kg   =   ?   g   answer _____

   (b)   55 g   =   ?   mg   answer _____

   (c)   72 mg   =   ?   mcg   answer _____

   (d)   105 L   =   ?   ml   answer _____

   (e)   48 m   =   ?   cm   answer _____

   (f)   1,257 mm   =   ?   m   answer _____

   (g)   387 cm   =   ?   mm   answer _____

   (h)   43 mm   =   ?   cm   answer _____

   (i)   982 mg   =   ?   g   answer _____

   (j)   3,389 mg   =   ?   kg   answer _____

   (k)   0.0765 mg   =   ?   mcg   answer _____

   (l)   0.00376 g   =   ?   µg   answer _____

   (m)   5,786 ml   =   ?   L   answer _____

   (n)   0.0698 L   =   ?   ml   answer _____

   (o)   0.00997 kg   =   ?   mg   answer _____

   (p)   8,023,766 g   =   ?   kg   answer _____

   (q)   7,569 mcg   =   ?   g   answer _____

   (r)   355.56 ml   =   ?   L   answer _____

   (s)   0.0298 m   =   ?   mm   answer _____

   (t)   0.002289 ml   =   ?   L   answer _____

   (u)   0.200897 kg   =   ?   mcg   answer _____

▼▼▼▼▼ *The answers to all problems can be found in the answer key starting on page 160.* ▼▼▼▼▼

If you had problems with Question 1, you need to review the previous material before continuing. If you are ready, then let's crank it up a notch and create some of the dreaded "word problems" using the metric system.

The best way to answer the following questions is to convert everything to the same units.

Example: 1 kg   +   300 g   = ?

Solution: (1,000 g + 300 g   = 1,300 g) *or* (1 kg + 0.3 kg = 1.3 kg)

PRACTICE

2. Yesterday I bought 3 cantaloupes of various weights. One weighed 635 g, another weighed 0.58 kg, and the third weighed 428,970 mg. How many grams did all three cantaloupes weigh?

   I like to convert all the units to whatever unit is asked for in the answer.

3. Yesterday I also purchased a really big bunch of white grapes weighing a whopping 1.27 kg. When I arrived home, I was so bored I decided to count each and every little grape. Guess what? There was a total of 429 grapes. How many grams did each grape weigh?

4. I was on a tear yesterday at the grocery store and also bought a pound of coffee. If a pound weighs 454 g, how many pots of coffee can be prepared if each pot requires 22,700 mg of ground coffee?

5. My daughter Angela loves Cranberry Juice Cocktail, so I bought her a bottle containing 64 fluid ounces. I noticed on the bottle next to the 64 fl oz there was also the number 1.89 L. Being the new resident expert with the metric system, I am sure you immediately recognized what the 1.89 L means, but could you tell me how many 210-ml glasses of juice Angela can get from the bottle?

6. The grocery store is only 2.6 kilometers from my home. How many meters would I travel in a round-trip to the store and back home?

7. Last summer I gained 8 pounds on vacation. How many kilograms would this be if there are 454 grams per pound?

(By now you are probably thinking I'm a geek and wouldn't have a weight problem if I'd "get a life" and quit counting grapes!)

8. My wife Patricia cut her finger. I noticed the bandage she used was 7.62 cm in length and the box contained 100 bandages. If I got very bored and decided to place the 99 remaining bandages end to end, how many meters would they stretch?

Now let's apply the metric system to pharmacy practice.

9. A pharmacy technician weighs four partially full bottles of salicylic acid. How many grams of salicylic acid does she have if the bottles contain 378 g, 0.86 kg, 198,000 mg, and 38,000,000 mcg?

10. A formula for a bulk salicylic acid ointment requires 1.5 kg of salicylic acid. You only have on hand the amount calculated in Question 9. How many additional milligrams of salicylic acid must you purchase?

11. How many 120-ml bottles can be filled from 3.84 L of a cough syrup?

12. A pharmacy buys 3 kg of flea powder and repackages it into powder "shaker" cans containing 90 g each. How many shakers could be *completely* filled with powder?

13. How many grams of thiamine HCl would be required to prepare 2500 capsules each containing 750 μg of thiamine HCl?

14. How many 30-mg codeine capsules can be prepared from 0.0009 kg of codeine?

15. If a vial contains 40 mg of tobramycin sulfate per milliliter, how many micrograms of tobramycin sulfate would be in 0.1 ml?

16. How many mm tall would a patient be who was measured at 178 cm?

▼▼▼▼▼ *The answers to all problems can be found in the answer key starting on page 160.* ▼▼▼▼▼

Apothecaries' System

At the beginning of this chapter, I mentioned the metric system was the primary and most recommended system of measurement used today. The apothecaries' system is antiquated but still occasionally appears in pharmacy and medical practice. This system measures weights and volumes, but it does not have a measure of length.

Although I do not recommend that you spend a lot of time in this section, it would behoove you to at least be familiar with the apothecaries' system so you can make conversions to the metric system whenever necessary.

The grain is the primary unit of weight in this system. The abbreviation for grain (gr) is frequently confused with the abbreviation for gram (g), but these weights are very different. The pound in this system is not the same as the 16-ounce pound you are familiar with in everyday life. This pound only has 12 ounces. The grain is the only weight in this system that you will see frequently in contemporary pharmacy practice. All of these weights are being replaced by the gram in the metric system.

APOTHECARIES' WEIGHTS

20 grains (gr)	=	1 scruple	℈		
3 scruples	=	1 dram	ʒ	=	60 grains
8 drams	=	1 ounce	℥	=	480 grains
12 ounces	=	1 pound		=	5,760 grains

APOTHECARIES' FLUID MEASURES

60 minims ♏	=	1 fluid dram	fʒ		
8 fluid drams	=	1 fluid ounce	f℥	=	480 minims
16 fluid ounces	=	1 pint	(pt.)		
2 pints	=	1 quart	(qt.)	=	32 fluid ounces
4 quarts (8 pints)	=	1 gallon	(gal.)	=	128 fluid ounces

Ounces, pints, quarts, and gallons are the measures of volume that most of you see in everyday life. They will eventually be replaced by the liter and milliliter of the metric system.

PRACTICE

17. Convert the following:

(a)   5 quarts   =   _____fluid ounces

(b)   3 gallons   =   _____pints

(c)   498 pints   =   _____gallons

(d)   322 fl. ounces   =   _____quarts

(e)   960 minims   =   _____fluid ounces

(f)   480 fl.drams   =   _____fluid ounces

(g)   1/4 gallon   =   _____pints

(h)   76 ounces   =   _____grains

(i)   64 drams   =   _____ounces

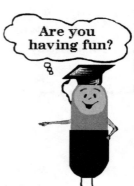

Are you having fun?

18. How many 4-fluid-ounce bottles can be filled from 2 gallons of elixir?

19. How many apothecaries' ounces would a patient receive in a week if she took 180 grains daily?

20. How many capsules containing $1\frac{3}{4}$ grains each of a drug can be prepared from $1\frac{3}{4}$ apothecaries' ounces of the drug?

▼▼▼▼▼ *The answers to all problems can be found in the answer key starting on page 160.* ▼▼▼▼▼

Avoirdupois System

*The avoirdupois system is another antiquated system used **only** for measuring weight. Even though it too is being replaced by the metric system of weights, you will find that you are already familiar with its units even though you probably cannot pronounce the name of this system!*

AVOIRDUPOIS WEIGHTS

1 ounce (oz)	=	437.5 grains (gr)	=	28.4 g
16 ounces	=	1 pound (lb)	=	7,000 gr

Did you notice what the apothecaries' and the avoirdupois systems of weight have in common? Of course you did. They both contain grains as the smallest unit.

Did you also notice that an ounce in one system has 437.5 gr and in the other 480 gr? The ounce and the pound in the avoirdupois system of weights are the ones you use every day. The apothecaries' ounces and pounds are rarely (if ever) used, so don't spend your life worrying too much about that system of weights.

Now let's try a few problems!

21. Convert the following:

   (a) 168 lb   = _____ oz   (d)   768 gr   = _____ lb

   (b) 137 oz   = _____ lb   (e)   1,276 gr   = _____ oz

   (c) 36 oz   = _____ gr

22. A pharmacy technician found three containers of bismuth subnitrate powder containing: $1\frac{1}{8}$ pound, 15 oz, and 3,276 gr. How many total ounces of bismuth subnitrate powder did she find?

NOW LET'S GO FIGURE OUT HOW TO RELATE
          ALL THESE CRAZY VALUES TO THE METRIC SYSTEM!

Common Conversion Factors

There are several conversion factors that will help you convert to the metric system when confronted with apothecaries' or avoirdupois values. I've rounded them off to keep you from going loony!

METRIC CONVERSIONS

WEIGHT			*VOLUME*

1 gram (g) = 15.4 grains (gr)

1 grain (gr) = 65 milligrams (mg) = 0.065 g

1 pound (lb) = 454 grams (g) = 0.454 kg

1 kilogram (kg) = 2.2 pounds (lb) ($\frac{1000}{454}$ = 2.2)

1 ounce (oz) = 28.4 g (454 g/16 = 28.4 g)

1 fluid ounce = 30 milliliters (ml)

1 pint (pt) = 16 fluid ounces = 480 ml

1 gallon = 3,840 milliliters (ml)

Many times you will notice on a pint bottle that the volume is 473 ml. Why then would I tell you to use 480 ml? The reason is the manufacturers are using the exact equivalents and I'm rounding off. In reality, a fluid ounce contains 29.57 ml and to calculate the volume of a pint you would multiply by 16, giving an answer of 473.12 ml per pint. So ask yourself, do you like my rounded off numbers or the real numbers? Most pharmacies will use the rounded off 480-ml conversion for a pint.

Household Equivalents

This last system of measurement has no real scientific basis. It was created to assist the patient with measuring while at home. Telling the average consumer to take "$\frac{1}{6}$ apothecaries' fluid ounce" of a cough syrup would be silly, and most patients wouldn't have a clue as to what you were saying. Instead, you can simply tell the patient to take 1 teaspoonful of the medication, and the patient will not only receive the correct dose but will smile and understand what you said.

This need for simple and accurate methods for measuring led to the evolution of household equivalents. There are many household equivalents (examples: dessert-spoonful, wine-glass,) but, as always, I will rescue you and only require you to learn the ones routinely seen in pharmacy practice.

1 teaspoonful (tsp)	=	5	milliliters (ml)
1 tablespoonful (tbsp)	=	15	milliliters (ml)
1 fluid ounce (oz) (f℥)	=	30	milliliters (ml)
1 pint (pt)	=	480	milliliters (ml)

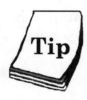

Always make sure patients use measuring devices when directions are given to take a "teaspoon" or "tablespoon" dose. Why? Because teaspoons range in size from approximately 3 ml all the way to 7 ml so there is great potential for error. Tablespoons can vary by almost 8 ml, which can also lead to significant problems in dosing.

Due to the use of household equivalents, many liquid medications are prepared to contain a certain quantity of a drug per teaspoonful (5 ml). Several examples of this are: amoxicillin 250 mg/5 ml and diphenhydramine 12.5 mg/5 ml. Physicians will tell the patient, in the case of the amoxicillin, to take "1 teaspoonful three times a day," and the patient will receive 250 mg in each dose. If a patient uses a 3-ml teaspoon instead of the measuring device, he would receive only 150 mg of the amoxicillin instead of the recommended 250-mg dose. **See how important you are?**

Question: How many teaspoons are in a tablespoon?

Answer: 3   (3 × 5 ml = 15 ml)

Question: How many tablespoons are in a pint?

Answer: 32   (480 ÷ 15 = 32)

PRACTICE

23. Convert the following:

(a)	4.5 teaspoons	=	_____ml
(b)	325 lb	=	_____kg
(c)	3,000 gr	=	_____g
(d)	289 kg	=	_____lb
(e)	75 ml	=	_____tsp
(f)	67 g	=	_____gr
(g)	6.5 lb	=	_____oz
(h)	118 mg	=	_____gr
(i)	727 oz	=	_____lb
(j)	1,700 ml	=	_____pt
(k)	43 gr	=	_____mg
(l)	35 tbsp	=	_____tsp
(m)	4.8 pints	=	_____ml
(n)	3 fluid ounces	=	_____tsp
(o)	64 fluid ounces	=	_____pints
(p)	111 kg	=	_____lb
(q)	485 lb	=	_____kg
(r)	4 quarts	=	_____liters
(s)	15,000 ml	=	_____gallons
(t)	$5\frac{3}{4}$ lb	=	_____g
(u)	2,150 ml	=	_____tbsp
(v)	$3\frac{1}{2}$ oz	=	_____g

Now let's put it all together. Good luck!

24. A pharmacist dispensed four prescriptions for a narcotic in the following quantities: 18 gr, 2,600 mg, 1.3 g, and $\frac{1}{4}$ avoirdupois ounce (oz).

(a) How many grains of narcotic were dispensed in all four prescriptions?

(b) How many mg of narcotic were dispensed in all four prescriptions?

(c) Prior to filling the four prescriptions, the pharmacy technician noted there was $\frac{1}{2}$ avoirdupois ounce (oz) of narcotic in stock. How many grams of narcotic remain after the four prescriptions have been filled?

25. A pharmacy technician prepared six prescriptions containing the following volumes: $\frac{1}{8}$ gallon, $\frac{1}{2}$ quart, $\frac{1}{2}$ pint, 5 fl.ounces, 8 tbsp, and 15 tsp.

(a) How many teaspoons were dispensed in the six prescriptions?

(b) If the pharmacy technician started with a gallon, how many milliliters remain after filling the six prescriptions?

▼▼▼▼▼ *The answers to all problems can be found in the answer key starting on page 160.* ▼▼▼▼▼

IF YOU HAVE MASTERED THE BASICS OF PHARMACY CALCULATIONS, IT IS TIME TO MOVE TO CHAPTER 3, THE MEAT AND TATERS OF THIS BOOK!

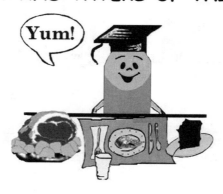
Yum!

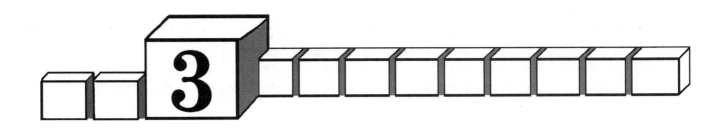

RATIO AND PROPORTION

*I*n my opinion, Chapter 3 is the key to understanding how to perform almost every type of math problem you will encounter in both pharmacy practice and in everyday life. Your success in future chapters will hinge on how well you master this section. Even calculations involving "drip rates," "milliequivalents," "percentages," and "reducing and enlarging formulas" will be done by the exact same process.

As I mentioned in the Preface, you do not need to know a lot of fancy math procedures to be successful with most medical and pharmacy calculations. This is easy material, but we will spend much more time than other textbooks do on ratio and proportion because I want you to really know this concept inside and out. By doing so, you will find pharmacy calculations are, as they say back home, a "piece of cake"!

OBJECTIVES

Upon mastery of Chapter 3 you will be able to:

Express common and decimal fractions as ratios.
Have an understanding of the process of ratio and proportion.
Solve problems using the process of ratio and proportion.

Back in Chapter 1, we discussed common fractions and decimals. Hopefully, you remember that the fraction $\frac{1}{2}$ is also equal to 0.5, but did you know that this can also be expressed as a percent and as a ratio? In this chapter, we will focus on ratios. Later in the book I will cover percents.

**So it's off to the
"ratio and proportion" races!**

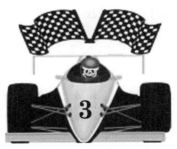

You know 0.5 is equal to $\frac{5}{10}$ and also that $\frac{5}{10}$ can be reduced all the way down to $\frac{1}{2}$ by simply dividing the numerator and denominator by the number 5. These two fractions ($\frac{1}{2}$ and $\frac{5}{10}$) are exactly equal in value with $\frac{1}{2}$ reduced to lowest terms.

Question: Are the fractions $\frac{3}{6}$, $\frac{4}{8}$, and $\frac{13}{26}$ also equal in value to $\frac{1}{2}$?

Answer: Yes, they are all equal. As an example, pull out your trusty calculator and let's take a look at $\frac{13}{26}$ which is the toughest one. Divide 13 by 26, and your answer should be 0.5 (if it isn't, you need to buy another calculator!). Try this same process with the other fractions, and you will continue to get 0.5 as an answer.

Question: What fraction of apples would be eaten if you bought a dozen and ate 6?

Answer: The answer is $\frac{6}{12}$ of the apples have been eaten. If you are really on a roll you probably said $\frac{1}{2}$ have been consumed. You may even have said 0.5 were eaten.

Question: What fraction of oranges are still good if you started with 16, and 12 of the oranges rotted before you could eat them?

Answer: In this case, we have $\frac{4}{16}$ of the oranges remaining. This can be reduced to $\frac{1}{4}$ simply by dividing the numerator and denominator by the common number 4. This means that $\frac{4}{16}$ is equal to $\frac{1}{4}$, which is also equal to 0.25.

The fraction of oranges that rotted is $\frac{12}{16}$ or $\frac{3}{4}$ or 0.75.

So What Is a Ratio?

Ratios are just a way of expressing the relationship of one quantity to another. When writing a ratio, you usually put a colon (:) between the numbers. Actually, a ratio is the same as a fraction, a percent, and even a decimal fraction.

I will not use ratios written with a colon very often in this text, but it is beneficial to have an understanding of the concept because you will sometimes encounter ratios in practice. We will discuss ratios in more depth in future chapters.

In most of the cases you will experience in pharmacy, the ratio indicates how much drug is in a solution.

Example: Epinephrine 1:1,000 solution

The epinephrine 1:1,000 solution indicates the amount of drug to the amount of total solution. This example means there is 1 part of epinephrine in 1,000 parts of solution.

The 1:1,000 ratio can also be written as $\frac{1}{1000}$ and 0.001.

Example: In the earlier question concerning apples, the ratio of eaten to total apples is 6:12 or 1:2 (when reduced). Do not get all caught up in this.
I will usually write the 1:2 as a fraction ($\frac{1}{2}$) and proceed from there.

Question: In the orange example, what is the ratio of edible oranges ?

Answer: 4:16, which is also the same as $\frac{4}{16}$ or $\frac{1}{4}$ or 1:4

NOW LET'S DO SOMETHING USEFUL
           WITH ALL OF THESE FRACTIONS!

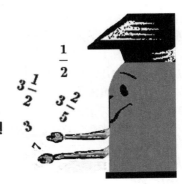

Proportion

A proportion is the expression of equality of two ratios or fractions to each other. For just a minute, I want you to think back to your pre-algebra coursework when you learned all that stuff about (A/B = C/D). Does that bring back bad memories? We are not going to venture beyond this simple equation for your sake and for mine, but it is important for you to understand the concept.

The equation (A/B = C/D) is actually a proportion where 2 equal fractions are put side by side. Let's set up a proportion based on our earlier discussion in this chapter by putting 2 equal fractions in a proportional equation. In the "apple" example, we said that $\frac{6}{12}$ was equal to $\frac{1}{2}$. To prepare a proportion, we simply put these fractions equal to each other just like this: ($\frac{1}{2} = \frac{6}{12}$). This is the same as (A/B = C/D).

So what! *Well, if in the "apple" example I had said only that you had 12 apples and ate $\frac{1}{2}$ of them, could you have told me how many were eaten? I bet you knew the answer was 6 without even solving it on paper. Am I correct? You actually performed a ratio and proportion problem in your cute little head and probably didn't know the process was actually taking place.*

Try another one. *If you have 24 eggs and break $\frac{1}{4}$ of them, how many did you break? There is a good chance you said 6 without thinking much about it. Or possibly you multiplied 24 times $\frac{1}{4}$ to get your answer, i.e., 24 x $\frac{1}{4}$ = 6.*

The process really doesn't get much harder, so stay focused on what is happening.

I want you to take a minute and solve the same problem by the process of ratio and proportion (A/B = C/D) → 1/4 = C/24. OOPS! I'm missing a number over 24. We already know that the "C" is equal to "6" making the equation $\frac{1}{4} = \frac{6}{24}$, and we know both fractions are equal, but what if the numbers were more complicated?

The overall process is very simple, but I believe it is best to learn with easy numbers and then advance to the more complex ones. By remembering easy-to-understand examples like those discussed so far, you will be able to go back to those examples if you become confused.

You probably remember your teachers telling you, "if you have the equation A/B = C/D and you know 3 of the numbers, you can solve for the missing 4th number." The method most people use (and the only one I will use) is cross multiplication. Simply multiply numerators times denominators, and solve for the missing number.

I like to use a question mark (?) for the "unknown" when solving ratio and proportion problems. Most people use an X, but I like the ?, because we will not confuse this sign with the "times" or "multiplying" symbol, i.e., " x." Now let's cross multiply and solve for an unknown.

Example: Using the previous "egg" question, solve for (?):

$$\frac{1}{4} = \frac{?}{24}$$

Step 1. Multiply numerators times denominators (1×24) and $(4 \times ?)$ and make them equal to each other.

(1×24) = $(4 \times ?)$

or

$(1)\,(24)$ = $(4)\,(?)$ **I like to solve these with this format.**

Step 2. Now solve for (?):

$(1)\,(24)$ = $(4)\,(?)$ *(Multiply the 1 times 24 to get 24.)*

24 = $(4)\,(?)$

$\frac{24}{4}$ = ? **This step is where many people make mistakes.**
You already knew that $\frac{1}{4}$ of 24 was 6, but now you know how to get there.

6 = ?

Now you try one.

Question: If a book has 68 pages, how many pages would there be in 30 of these books?

Solution: **Step 1.** Set up these two fractions equal to each other.
1 **book**/68 **pages** = 30 **books**/(?)

Step 2. *Cross* multiply numerators times denominators.
1 **book**/68 **pages** = 30 **books**/(?)

(68 **pages**)(30 **books**) = (1 **book**) (?)

2,040 **pages** (**books**) = 1 **book** (?)

Step 3. Divide and solve for (?).
2,040 **pages** (**books**)/1 **book** = ?

2,040 **pages** = ?

The "book" units cancel when you divide, giving an answer in "pages."

PLEASE STOP RIGHT HERE!

Before we go any further, I want to ask you a question, and **I want you to be honest. Did you estimate the answer to the last question?**

Your response is most likely *NO* if you are like the majority of my students and most practitioners. If you said *YES*, then you get a gold star, and I apologize for jumping on your case. As I mentioned earlier, you can avoid many "stupid" errors by simply estimating answers. In the last question, you could have easily said 70 pages times 30 books equals 2100. (I know there were 68 pages, but you are just rounding off and making a guesstimate of the correct answer.) What frequently happens in ratio and proportion is that people will divide by the wrong number and get a ridiculous answer. In the last example, if you divided 68 by 30 you would get an answer of 2.27 pages. Now does that make a lot of sense? For the record, I would include 2.27 as a choice in a multiple choice question to catch the "meatheads" who do not think and just start working problems without estimating.

Please take my word that you will be a better pharmacy technician or any other type of professional if you just think a little before you act. This estimation process takes practice, but it should only take about 3–5 seconds per problem and is well worth the time and effort.

OK, OK, enough lecturing. Let's get back to work!

Question: If 12 fishing hooks cost $1.25, how much will 20 cost?

Solution:

12 **hooks**/$1.25	=	20 **hooks**/?	(*set up proportion*)
(12 **hooks**) (?)	=	($1.25) (20 **hooks**)	(*cross multiply*)
12 **hooks** (?)	=	$ 25 **hooks**	
?	=	$ 25 **hooks**/12 **hooks**	(*solve for ?*)
?	=	$ 2.08	

("Hooks" cancel when you divide, leaving your answer in dollars.)

I would estimate before solving this problem that since 12 hooks cost $1.25, 24 would cost about $2.50. (Since you want the price of 20 hooks, the answer will be less than $2.50.)

PLEASE STOP AGAIN!!!

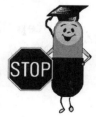

All right, I've got one more question for you. **Are you looking at the answers before working the questions or just skipping the "easy" stuff?**

Please work every problem in this book so you get the full benefit.   P.S. I'm sorry for jumping on your case if you are in the 5% of people who work in a methodical manner.

Now let's have some fun!

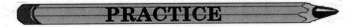

PRACTICE

Please work all problems in your book before checking answers.

1. Solve for the equivalent fractions, decimals, and ratio forms for the following and reduce to lowest terms when necessary.

	Fraction	Decimal	Ratio
(a)	$\frac{4}{12}$	_____	_____
(b)	$\frac{20}{210}$	_____	_____
(c)	$\frac{38}{218}$	_____	_____
(d)	_____	0.6	_____
(e)	_____	0.005	_____
(f)	_____	0.44	_____
(g)	_____	_____	3:15
(h)	_____	_____	30:600
(i)	_____	_____	600:2,400

2. How many calories are in a 19-ounce box of Frosted Mini-Wheats® if there are 200 calories per serving? (A serving is 2.1 ounces.)

3. How many shampoos can I get out of a 750-ml bottle of Pert Plus® shampoo if I use approximately 1 teaspoonful of this product per shampoo? **An advantage of being bald like me is that you don't need much shampoo!**

4. My daughter Kim teaches and notes that the average student uses 75 sheets of paper every week.

   (a)   How many sheets will a student use in a 42-week school year?

   (b)   How many sheets will a class of 26 students use in a week?

5. A Diet Sprite® contains 2.92 mg of sodium per fluid ounce. How many grams of sodium are contained in a 12-ounce can?

   I'm trying to trick you with this question. See if you can beat me on this one.

6. My son Bill recently went to Central America for his honeymoon. While on this trip, he wanted to purchase his "honey" a gold bracelet that cost 480,000 *rumples*. (I really don't remember the correct currency name, but *rumples* sounds good enough for this question.) How much in American currency did the bracelet cost? *(1,500 rumples = $1)*

7. My baby daughter Abby goes through an average of 1 Pamper® diaper every 2 hours. How many diapers will we need to buy for a two-week vacation?

   (It is difficult to relax on a vacation and change that many diapers!)

8. If your car gets 18 miles per gallon of gasoline, how many pints of gas will you need to take a 698-mile trip?

9. Coppertone Sport® Ultra Sweatproof - SPF 15 dry lotion contains 1.2 mg of octylmethoxycinnamate per fluid ounce. How many micrograms of this chemical would be in $\frac{1}{2}$ pint of the sunblock lotion?

10. If you can fill one prescription every 135 seconds, how many prescriptions could you fill every hour? **(Assuming no phone interruptions, lunch or bathroom breaks, or whiney patients!)**

11. A manufacturer wants to prepare 500,000 diazepam tablets containing 5 mg of diazepam each. How many kilograms of diazepam will be required to prepare this batch?

12. If a drug contains 25 mg of an expectorant per tablespoon, how much expectorant would be in a quart of this medication?

13. How much would 3 lb of sulfur cost if you purchased 182 lb of sulfur for $2,134?

14. An antiflatulent medication contains 20 mg of simethicone per infant dose of 0.3 ml. How many grams of simethicone are contained in a 1-fluid-ounce bottle?

15. The average aspirin tablet contains 5 grains of acetylsalicylic acid (ASA). How many grams of ASA would be in a 250-tablet bottle of aspirin?

16. A pharmacy technician prepared a large batch of zinc oxide ointment containing 10 grams of zinc oxide in every 100 grams of ointment. How much ointment was prepared if the technician used $\frac{3}{8}$ lb of zinc oxide?

17. A patient weighs 186 pounds and the dosing schedule for a medication is given for weight measured in kilograms. How many kilograms would you calculate the patient weighs?

18. If an alprazolam tablet contains 0.25 mg of active ingredient, how many grains would be contained in a 100-tablet bottle?

19. A pint of cough medicine contains 960 mg of an antitussive medication. How many grams of the medication would be in a 2-teaspoonful dose?

20. How many milligrams of nitroglycerin would be contained in 30 tablets each containing $\frac{1}{150}$ gr of nitroglycerin?

21. If a patient receives 1.4 ml of 5% dextrose intravenous solution per minute, how many liters of solution would the patient receive in a day?

22. An injectable product contains 750 mcg per vial. How many vials would be needed to provide a 15-mg dose?

23. If green soap tincture costs $32.00 per gallon, how much would a liter cost?

24. A pharmacy technician prepares 3 liters of syrup using 5 lb of sugar. How many grams of sugar would be in a teaspoonful of the syrup?

25. If 2 grains of phenobarbital are divided into 90 capsules, how many μg of phenobarbital would be in each capsule?

▼▼▼▼▼ *The answers to all problems can be found in the answer key starting on page 160.* ▼▼▼▼▼

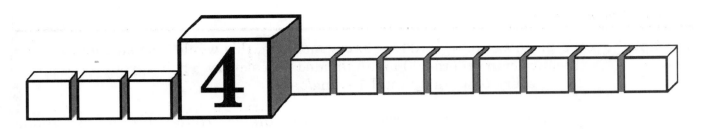

INTERPRETING DRUG ORDERS
AND
CALCULATING DOSES

In Chapter 4, we will take all your skills from the first three chapters and apply them in calculating doses of medications. Before you start doing the math, you must first learn a few more "foundation" skills.

At the beginning of this chapter, you will learn how to interpret a written drug order. Later we will work some calculations related to drug orders. I have some great news for you. The math is exactly like the ratio and proportion questions you did in Chapter 3. I will just change the questions a little to relate more to individual patients.

OBJECTIVES

Upon mastery of Chapter 4 you will be able to:

Write standard medical abbreviations.
Read medical notations and determine a dosage regimen.
Calculate appropriate doses for patients.
Perform flow rate calculations.
Solve for a dose using Body Surface Area (BSA).
Determine appropriate doses for chemotherapy using BSA.

The terms dose and dosage warrant clarification, so you know what I'm talking about.

*A **dose** is the quantity of a drug taken by a patient. It may be expressed as a "daily" dose, "single" dose, or even a "total" dose, which refers to all the drug taken throughout therapy. A "daily" dose may be given once daily, which is a "single" daily dose, or it can be divided throughout the day and would then be known as a "divided" dose.*

Example: If a physician orders 100 mg every morning, this would be a single dose. If the physician orders 100 mg in divided doses every 6 hours, you would give 25 mg every 6 hours (to total 100 mg/day).

Doses vary tremendously due to differences in drug potency, routes of administration, and the patient's age, weight, protein binding, and kidney and liver function. Many factors enter into establishing a correct dose, and many dispensing errors are related either to giving the wrong dose or misinterpreting an order.

As a pharmacy technician, you can contribute greatly to patient care by being able to calculate doses and read medication "orders." By having these skills, you will eventually catch mistakes that have been overlooked by other healthcare providers. So if you want to be the best technician in town, learn appropriate doses and dosage regimens and don't be afraid to speak up if you spot an error.

A **dosage regimen** *refers to the schedule of medication administration. Here's a possible regimen you might encounter.*

Example: If a physician orders 250 mg every 6 hours, the *dose* is 250 mg and the *dosage regimen* is "every 6 hours."

Read this

In many pharmacy calculation textbooks you will encounter a truckload of rules for calculating doses. Names for some of these rules include: Young's rule, Clark's rule, Fried's rule, Cowling's rule. Unfortunately, these rules treat children and infants as just "little adults" with no consideration to any other physiological factors. Do not use them under any circumstances.

I have *never* seen anyone use these rules to dose. In every case you will encounter, appropriate doses will be specified by the manufacturer in the package inserts. Suitable doses can also be found in numerous references such as the *Physicians' Desk Reference* (PDR), the *USP DI - Volume I, Drug Facts and Comparisons*, and others. Doses are listed according to age and are given in milligrams or milliliters per kilogram or pound of body weight.

All you need to know to calculate doses is our friend ratio and proportion.

Before we start learning abbreviations, you need to know about one more thing —the drug order— the "bread and butter" of what gives you a job as a pharmacy technician.

You are going to be mad at me now! Guess what?

Now you need to take a lot of time and memorize all of the following abbreviations, all of which you will encounter frequently in routine pharmacy practice.

Please do not continue before learning these.

COMMON MEDICAL ABBREVIATIONS

FREQUENCY

a.c.	before meals		p.c.	after meals
a.m.	morning		h.s.	at bedtime
p.m.	afternoon or evening		q.d.	once daily
ad. lib.	as desired		stat	immediately
p.r.n.	as needed		q.o.d.	every other day
b.i.d.	twice a day		t.i.d.	three times a day
q.i.d.	four times a day		min.	minute
h. or hr.	hour		q.h.	every hour
q.2h	every 2 hours		q.8h	every 8 hours
q.12h	every 12 hours (etc. for all hours)		u.d.	as directed

ROUTE

a.d.	right ear		a.s.	left ear
a.u.	both ears		IM	intramuscular
inj.	injection		IV	intravenous
IVPB	intravenous piggyback		IVP	intravenous push
o.d.	right eye		o.u.	both eyes
o.s. or o.l.	left eye		p.o.	by mouth
pr	per rectum		SL	sublingual
SC or SQ	subcutaneous		ID	intradermal

DOSAGE FORMS

aq.	aqueous (water)		cap	capsule
comp.	compound		gtt.	drop
pulv	powder		sol.	solution
supp.	suppository		susp.	suspension
syr.	syrup		tab	tablet
tinct or tr	tincture		ung	ointment

MISCELLANEOUS

a	before		p	after
c	with		s	without
q	every		ad	up to
aa	of each		ante	before
DC, d/c, or disc.	discontinue		dil.	dilute
disp.	dispense		div.	divide
d.t.d.	give of such doses		dx	diagnosis
et	and		ft.	make
N/V	nausea and vomiting		hx	history
q.s.	a sufficient quantity		rt.	right
non rep. or N.R.	do not repeat		GI	gastrointestinal
R/O	ruled out		noct.	night
NPO	nothing by mouth		Sig	write on label
SOB	shortness of breath		BP	blood pressure
UTI	urinary tract infection		M	mix
URI	upper respiratory infection		HA	headache

The **drug order** consists of seven parts that should always be present. Many state Boards of Pharmacy require additional information, but the following are the "biggies" you must know to correctly fill a prescription:

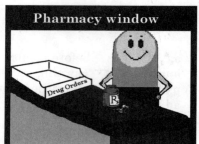

☐   Name of the patient to receive the medication.
☐   Name of the drug to be dispensed or administered.
☐   Dose of the drug.
☐   Route by which the drug is to be taken or administered.
☐   Dosage regimen by which the drug is to be taken or administered.
☐   Date (and time in institutional settings) when the order was written.
☐   Signature of the person writing the order or prescription.

Note   Prescriptions and drug orders differ in that drug orders are utilized in institutions and prescriptions are used in outpatient (community) settings. The legal requirements vary with each of these methods by which practitioners communicate medication requests.

Example: Prescription:
Ampicillin 250 mg caps.
Sig.   i cap. p.o. q.i.d.

"Sig." means to type on label the following: Take 1 capsule by mouth 4 times a day.

Example: Physician's drug order:
Demerol® 50 mg IM q.2-3h p.r.n. pain

For this order, the nurse would administer 50 mg of Demerol® intramuscularly every 2 to 3 hours as needed for pain.

Question: Now write down what the following prescription means.
                                    (don't peek at the answer).
Reglan 10 mg
i tab. p.o., q.i.d., a.c. and h.s.

Answer: Take 1 tablet by mouth, four times a day, before meals and at bedtime.

Body Surface Area (BSA)

*One last topic in the area of dosing you need to be familiar with is **body surface area**, also referred to as BSA. This procedure uses a patient's volume rather than weight. It is frequently used with patients receiving chemotherapy and sometimes with children. Body surface area is measured in square meters (m^2); most of the dosing we will see is in milligrams per square meter (mg/m^2). These problems are also solved by ratio and proportion. Just substitute the appropriate BSA for weight in our equation.*

But how do I solve for the body surface area?

See the following nomograms for the determination of BSA. Please note that there is a nomogram for children (page 48) and one for adults (page 49). To solve for BSA, there are five steps.

Step 1.	Make sure you are looking at the correct nomogram, i.e., adult or child.
Step 2.	Place a dot on the patient's weight on the vertical line to the right.
Step 3.	Place a dot on the patient's height on the vertical line to the left.
Step 4.	Connect the dots by drawing a line with a straight edge.
Step 5.	Read the patient's BSA, located on the center vertical line at the intersection where the line you drew in **Step 4** intersects.

Question: What is the BSA for a child who is 32 inches tall and weighs 45 pounds?

Answer: Make sure you are using the *child* nomogram, and place dots on the 32-inch mark (left column) and on the 45-lb mark (right column). Connect the dots with a straight line. The BSA of 0.63 m^2 for this child is located on the center line.

Question: What is the BSA for a 52-year-old man who is 170-cm tall and weighs 70 kg?

Answer: Use the *adult* nomogram. The BSA for this patient is approximately 1.8 m^2.

Question: What would be the dose of a medication for the child in the first question if the medication is normally dosed at 50 mg/m^2?

Answer: Solve by ratio and proportion: 50 **mg**/1 **m²** = ?/0.63 **m²**
                                        31.5 **mg** = ? (the child's dose)

Question: What would be the dose in micrograms if the dose of a drug for the 52-year-old man in the second question is 0.04 mg/m^2 ?

Answer: Change the dose to mcg at the beginning to make this easier, i.e., 40 mcg.
                    40 **mcg**/1 **m²** = ?/1.8 **m²**
                    72 **mcg** = ? (the patient's dose)

NOMOGRAM FOR CHILDREN
Determination of body surface from height and mass[1]

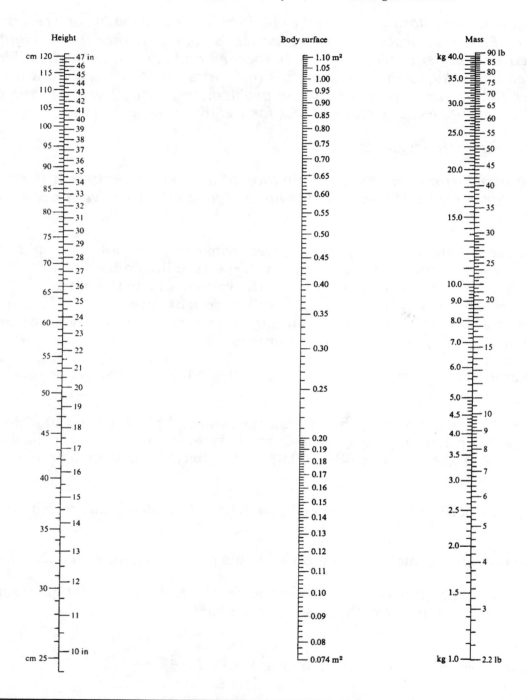

[1] From the formula of Du Bois and Du Bois, *Arch Intern Med,* 17, 863 (1916): $S = M^{0.425} \times H^{0.725} \times 71.84$, or $\log S = \log M \times 0.425 + \log H \times 0.725 + 1.8564$ (S = body surface in cm^2, M = mass in kg, H = height in cm).

Source: C. Lentner, Ed., *Geigy Scientific Tables,* 8th ed, vol 1, Basel: Ciba-Geigy; 1981: 226–7.

NOMOGRAM FOR ADULTS
Determination of body surface from height and mass[1]

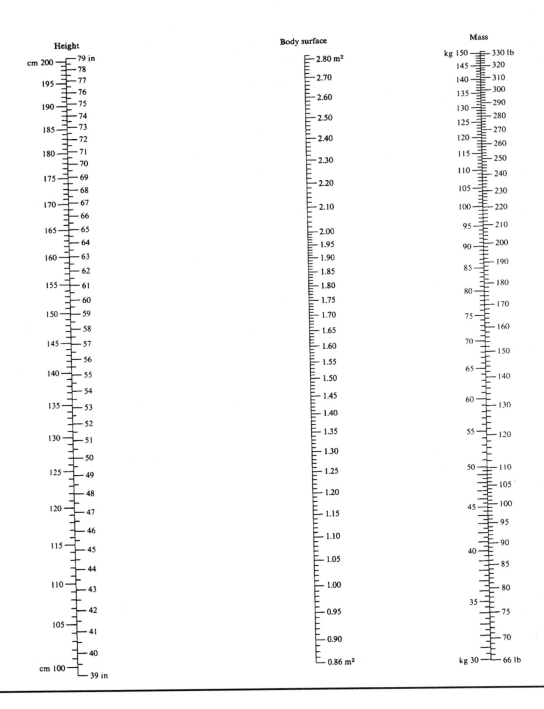

[1] From the formula of Du Bois and Du Bois, *Arch Intern Med,* 17, 863 (1916): $S = M^{0.425} \times H^{0.725} \times 71.84$, or $\log S = \log M \times 0.425 + \log H \times 0.725 + 1.8564$ (S = body surface in cm^2, M = mass in kg, H = height in cm).

Source: C. Lentner, Ed., *Geigy Scientific Tables,* 8th ed, vol 1,
Basel: Ciba-Geigy; 1981: 226–7.

Chemotherapy Dosing

In the last section, I mentioned that the body surface area (BSA) method of calculating doses is frequently used for cancer patients receiving chemotherapy. There are many safety considerations that must be taken into account in prescribing, compounding, and administering antineoplastic drugs. It is beyond the scope of this textbook to discuss these issues, but you need to be aware that specialized training is required for handling many chemotherapy products. Now let's solve for chemotherapy doses utilizing the body surface area method.

Example: Paclitaxel is an antineoplastic drug used in the treatment of various carcinomas, including ovarian and breast cancer. How many milligrams of paclitaxel would a 42-year-old, 131-lb, 65-inch tall female receive if the intravenous adult dose for breast carcinoma is 175 mg per square meter of body surface area repeated every twenty-one days?

Solution: Utilizing the nomogram for *adults*, the BSA is approximately 1.65 m². Now plug in your numbers and perform a ratio and proportion.
175 mg paclitaxel/1 m² = ?/1.65 m²   ? = 289 mg paclitaxel

Now you try one.

Question: Doxorubicin is an antineoplastic drug with many indications, including leukemia, carcinomas, and lymphomas. How many milligrams of doxorubicin would be administered in a single dose to a 20-kg, 96-cm child with leukemia if the intravenous dose is 30 mg per square meter of body surface area daily on 3 successive days every 4 weeks?

Answer: Utilizing the nomogram for *children*, the BSA is approximately 0.7 m².
30 mg doxorubicin/1 m² = ?/0.7 m²   ? = 21 mg doxorubicin

Question: How many milliliters of doxorubicin 2 mg/ml should be administered to provide the 4-week dosage regimen based on the *daily* dose you just calculated?

Answer: 2 mg doxorubicin/1 ml = 21 mg / ?   ? = 10.5 ml *per day*

10.5 ml/1 day = ?/3 days   ? = 31.5 ml every 4 weeks

PRACTICE

1. Interpret the following medication orders/prescription Sigs:

   (a) gtt iii o.d. q.6h, prn pain

   (b) tab i SL prn SOB

   (c) caps ii p.o. p.c. and h.s.

   (d) Humulin R® insulin 5 units SC stat

   (e) Ancef® 1 g IVPB q.6h

   (f) Inderal® 10mg p.o., q.i.d.

   (g) Dalmane® 15mg, cap. i, p.o., h.s.

   (h) Atrovent® inhaler, ii puffs, q.i.d., u.d.

   (i) Cortisporin Otic® gtt ii a.u. tid

   (j) Cefzil® 250mg/5mls   i tsp bid X 10 d

   (k) Persantine® 50mg, ii tabs q.i.d., 30 min a.c.

2. Without looking back, name the seven parts of a drug order.

   (a)

   (b)

   (c)

   (d)

   (e)

   (f)

   (g)

Questions 3–25 can all be worked by simple ratio and proportion.

3. A patient is to receive a prescription for tetracycline 250-mg capsules and the Sig. is caps. i p.o. qid x 10 days. How many capsules should be dispensed?

4. If the normal dose of a drug is 200 mcg, how many doses can be given from a multiple-dose vial containing 0.03 g of the drug?

5. If a patient takes diazepam 2 mg, t.i.d. for 30 days, how many grams of diazepam will the patient receive after 30 days of therapy?

6. If you gave a patient a 4-fluid-ounce bottle of cough syrup and it lasted six days, how many teaspoons of the syrup did the patient take each day?

7. How many milligrams of codeine would be in a tablespoonful of a medication containing 0.36 g of codeine in a 6-fluid-ounce bottle?

8. How many milliliters of digoxin elixir containing 50 mcg/ml would provide a 0.5-mg dose?

9. A beclomethasone inhaler provides 200 inhalations, and each inhalation contains 50 µg of the medication. How many milligrams of beclomethasone would be contained in an inhaler?

10. How many milliliters of amoxicillin 125 mg/5 ml should be dispensed to a patient if the Sig. reads: 1 tsp, po, t.i.d. x 10 days?

11. How many milliliters of an injection containing 0.2 mg/ml of a drug would provide a 125-mcg dose?

12. If a patient purchases 2-pint bottles of antacid and takes 2 tablespoonfuls every 6 hours, how many days will the antacid last?

13. An antitussive product contains 0.05 g of dextromethorphan in each teaspoonful dose. How many milligrams of dextromethorphan would be contained in a 4-ounce bottle?

14. How many units of heparin would a patient receive in a 24-hour period if she receives 20 ml of a heparin solution containing 50 units per ml every hour?

15. Regular U-100 insulin contains 100 units of insulin per ml. If a patient administers 10 units of insulin q.i.d., how many days will a 10-ml vial last?

16. How many milligrams of phenytoin would a 36-lb child receive if the physician wants the child to receive 3 mg of phenytoin per kg of body weight?

17. In Question 16, how many milliliters of a phenytoin suspension containing 30 mg/5 ml should the child receive?

18. How many 500-mg capsules of an antibiotic are needed to provide a dose of 25 mg/kg/day for a week for a patient weighing 220 lb?

19. If a 4-year-old accidentally ingested forty-two, 5-grain acetaminophen tablets, how many milligrams did the child ingest?

20. If the child in Question 19 weighed 44 lb, how much acetaminophen did the child ingest on a milligram-per-kilogram basis?

21. A patient routinely uses her metaproterenol inhaler six times a day and normally takes two puffs each time. How many canisters of this medication should she take with her on a 42-day vacation in Europe?

About 200 inhalations delivered per canister. | Hint |

22. If the dose of a medication for an infant is 2 mg/lb/day, how much would a 4-kg baby receive in 5 days?

23. A patient received a prescription for cefaclor suspension 125 mg/5 ml. The physician failed to write a quantity to be dispensed on the prescription. According to the following directions, how many ounces should be dispensed? Cefaclor 125/5
(Sig. 2 tsp, po, tid x 3d then 1 tsp, tid x 4d.)

24. If you were to prepare a liter of an elixir that is to contain 400 mcg of an alkaloid-per-tablespoonful dose, how many milligrams of the alkaloid would you need to use?

25. If the cost of a compounded prescription is $78.50 for a quart, how much would a ½-fluid-ounce dose cost?

▼▼▼▼▼ *The answers to all problems can be found in the answer key starting on page 160.* ▼▼▼▼▼

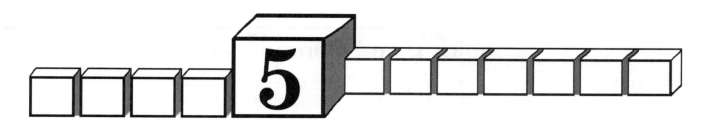

REDUCING AND ENLARGING FORMULAS AND COMPOUNDING

*I*n previous chapters, I mentioned on several occasions the term **compounded** pre-scriptions. When I use this term, I am talking about prescriptions that are extemporaneously prepared in the pharmacy.

The term **extemporaneous** basically means spontaneous. These are products that pharmacists and pharmacy technicians prepare themselves, unlike the majority of prescriptions that are made by pharmaceutical manufacturing companies.

OBJECTIVES

Upon mastery of Chapter 5 you will be able to:

Understand recipes for compounded prescriptions.
Solve for the quantities required to compound a prescription.
Enlarge a preexisting formula.
Reduce a preexisting formula.
Find volumes needed to compound a hyperalimentation solution.

In years past, most prescriptions were compounded in the pharmacy, but in the latter part of the 20th century the art (and need) for extemporaneous compounding declined significantly. Suddenly in the 1990's, there was a huge increase in the number of prescriptions that were being compounded in pharmacies. This increase was due to changes in regulations and due to a need for more specialized and individualized pharmaceutical products that were not available from pharmaceutical manufacturers.

These products range from vaginal suppositories, dermatological ointments and creams, tablets, capsules, sterile dosage forms, and much more. In this chapter, you will learn how to interpret a prescription for compounded products and how to reduce and enlarge preexisting formulas to meet your needs.

I believe the easiest way to teach the basics of compounding is by giving you different formulas as examples and following them with short discussions.
                                                        So let's go!

Cooking and Compounding

Example
1

Dry rice	1 cup
Water	2 cups
Salt	$\frac{1}{2}$ tsp
Margarine	1 tbsp

Combine water, salt, and margarine, and bring to a boil. Add rice to boiling water, reduce heat, cover, and simmer 20 minutes.   ***Makes 4 servings.***

I bet you have made something similar to this compounded product. Most of us refer to it as just plain old "rice." You simply measure the different components in the formula (recipe), and mix according to the directions to make 4 servings of rice.

Question: Let's pretend you are having company over tonight and need to prepare 8 servings instead of the 4 servings this recipe makes. How much dry rice would you need to prepare the 8 servings?

Answer: You probably said 2 cups of rice because you know from experience to double the formula to get twice the amount of cooked rice. You are exactly correct with your answer, but were you aware you were actually subconsciously performing a ratio and proportion? Think about the solution this way:

$$1 \text{ cup dry rice/4 servings} = \frac{?}{8} \text{ servings}$$

Looks Strangely Familiar, Doesn't It!

This technique can be used for all the components in the rice recipe, but there is a quicker method for enlarging a complete formula. Just take the amount you need (8 servings in this case) and divide it by the number of servings in the original formula (4). This will give you a factor of "2." Now just multiply everything in the recipe by "2" to get twice as many servings.
        (For you amateur cooks, you still simmer it for only 20 minutes, not 40!)

Guess what?
You have just mastered the skill known as enlarging formulas.

I told you this would be easy. In addition to learning how to enlarge a formula, you have already become familiar with interpreting a given recipe. By the way, did you know there is a lot of debate about the origin of the "Rx" symbol you see on prescriptions? Many people say it stands for the word "recipe," but there are other interpretations dating back to early Greek mythology. Just thought you might want to know.

Example
2

Fruit Cobbler

Biscuit baking mix	2 cups
Canned fruit pie filling	42 oz.
Skim milk	$\frac{3}{4}$ cup
Sugar	$\frac{1}{3}$ cup
Almond extract	$\frac{1}{4}$ tsp

Heat oven to 375 degrees. *Pour* fruit into 7" x 11" pan. *Mix* remaining ingredients. *Drop* dough by small spoonfuls on fruit. *Bake* 22 to 25 minutes or until golden. *Brush* with skim milk and top with sugar and cinnamon.
Makes 9 servings.

This example is similar to Example 1 in that it is very clear what quantities are needed to prepare the Fruit Cobbler, but I have another question for you.

Question: I'm home alone and have an incredible urge to make a small cobbler just for me. I look at the recipe and notice it is a formula for a cobbler big enough to feed 9 people. What factor would I multiply everything by to make a "mini" cobbler big enough to feed only 3 people? **I eat a lot!**

Answer: To get the conversion "factor," perform the calculations in the same manner as in Example 1. Just divide the servings you need (3) by the servings in the the formula (9).

$$\frac{3}{9} = 0.333$$

Your new factor is **0.333** *or* $\frac{1}{3}$. Now multiply each component in the formula by $\frac{1}{3}$ to get the new formula for a "mini" cobbler.

 Tip Don't forget that you can simply do a ratio and proportion if you only need to know one component. For example, to solve for the amount of fruit in 3 servings:

$$\frac{42\,oz.}{9\,Servings} = \frac{?}{3\,Servings}$$

You have mastered yet another skill, one known as reducing formulas. Now let's take a look at more "pharmacy" related examples and questions.

Example
3

Zinc oxide	50 g
Pine tar	120 g
Petrolatum	284 g

The ointment will contain 50 g of zinc oxide, 120 g of pine tar, and 284 g of petrolatum. If you *add* all the components together, you will have a *final* product weighing 454 g (i.e., 1 lb). Doesn't this look just like Examples 1 and 2?

Question: **Try to work this without looking at the solution.** How much pine tar would be required to prepare 1 kg of the ointment?

Solution: In this case, we are *enlarging* the formula to 1,000 g (i.e., 1 kg) from the original formula of 454 g (i.e., 1 lb).

120 g pine tar/454 g ointment = ?/1,000 g ointment
264.3 g pine tar = ?

You could also have taken the amount you need to make (1,000 g) and divide it by the total grams in the original formula (454 g) to get a factor of 2.2. You can then multiply the factor times 120 to get an answer of 264 g pine tar.

2.2 × 120 g = 264 g pine tar

In future problems, I will have you solve for only one component of the formula. I recommend you utilize the ratio and proportion approach because that is how I solve the answers. In real life, you will want to solve for a "factor" to expedite the math process.

Question: How much zinc oxide would be in 100 g of the ointment in Example 3?

Answer: 50 g zinc oxide/454 g ointment = ?/100 g ointment
11 g zinc oxide = ?

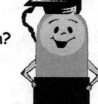

Did you estimate your answer or did I catch you again?

Example 4

Zinc oxide	50
Pine tar	120
Petrolatum	q.s. ad. 284

At first glance, this recipe looks very similar to Example 3, but there are two significant differences. First, there are no units listed next to the numbers. Whenever you are compounding with *solids* and the units are not included, this usually means to use *grams*, but always double check just in case it was a careless omission. The prescriber should always include the units when ordering a compounded prescription to avoid any possible mistakes. When units are not included with *liquids,* it usually means *milliliters*, but again check to make sure this is what the prescriber wanted.

The second big difference is the abbreviations (q.s. and ad.). The abbreviation **"q.s."** means "a sufficient quantity to make" and the abbreviation **"ad."** means to "add up to."

You will often see just one of these abbreviations, which in my opinion is plenty enough, but for some crazy reason people like to use both as I have in Example 4.

The abbreviations ad. and/or q.s. completely alter this formula from the recipe in Example 3. In Example 3, we added all the chemicals together to get a formula weight of 454 grams. In Example 4, the *final* weight is 284 grams because the ad. and/or q.s. indicate that you will *add enough petrolatum to make a final weight of 284 g.*

Question: How much petrolatum would be required to compound the prescription in Example 4?

Solution: If you have 50 grams of zinc oxide and 120 grams of pine tar, then your weight is already 170 grams with just those two components. If the final weight is to be 284 grams, then simply subtract the 170 grams from 284 grams and you will need 114 grams of petrolatum. To check your answer, add everything together and see if it all adds up to 284 grams.

CHECK: *120 g*
             50 g
      +114 g
         284 g   total weight

 To reduce or enlarge formulas, consider the total weight of this formula to be 284 grams, not 454 grams, as in Example 3.

Example 5

Benzyl benzoate	250	ml
Triethanolamine	5	ml
Oleic acid	20	ml
Purified water, to make	1000	ml

In this recipe, the words "to make" next to the purified water mean the same thing as using the abbreviation "q.s." In other words, the *final* volume will be 1000 ml. When working with liquids, you can measure all the volumes separately, but it is difficult to predict the final volume when you *add* all of them together.

For example, it is possible to add 20 ml of one chemical to 30 ml of another and wind up with a final volume of possibly 45–55 ml. This is due to factors you need not waste brain cells learning about, but you can have volume contractions and expansions. With this in mind, you would put the 250 ml of oleic acid, the 5 ml of triethanolamine, and the 20 ml of oleic acid together in a 1000-ml bottle and *add enough water to make* 1000 ml.

To reduce or enlarge this formula, use 1000 ml as the total volume.

Question: How much benzyl benzoate would be required to prepare a pint of the lotion in Example 5?

Answer: 250 ml benzyl benzoate/1000 ml lotion   =   ?/480 ml lotion
                      120 ml benzyl benzoate   =   ?

Note

Hopefully, you estimated the answer to be about half of the 250 ml.

Question: How much water would you use in compounding this recipe if the words "to make" were not in the formula?

Answer: You would measure 1000 ml of water and add it to the other components of the recipe. In this case, your final volume is going to be well above the 1000 ml you observed in Example 5.

Example 6

Camphor
Menthol   aa   1 g
Talc   100 g

This is probably the most *ridiculous* abbreviation of all! The "aa" in this prescription means "of each," which instructs you to use 1 gram of menthol and 1 gram of camphor. You will rarely see this, but I want you to recognize it in case it pops up. The reason I think this is a stupid abbreviation is because it takes no more effort to write 1 g than it takes to write aa, so why complicate an easy process!

Question: How much will the compound in Example 6 weigh?

Answer: 1 g camphor + 1 g menthol + 100 g talc = *102 grams*

Example 7

Phenobarbital   0.03 g
ASA   0.6 g
Lactose   qs
D.T.D.   caps. #30

In this prescription, the abbreviation "D.T.D." means "give of such doses." This means you are to prepare 30 capsules, with each capsule containing 600 mg of aspirin and 30 mg of phenobarbital. The qs next to the lactose means to add whatever quantity of lactose that is necessary to fill all the capsules. *(Capsules vary in size.)*

Example 8

Phenobarbital   0.9 g
ASA   18 g
Lactose   qs
M. ft. caps no. 30

Here "M. ft." means to "mix and make" 30 capsules from the total weight of the two drugs, i.e., divide the quantities in the recipe by 30 to get the amount in each capsule.

CAUTION: Always check whenever you have a question concerning a formula or a prescription, especially when you are unsure about the safety of a prescribed dose. With experience, you will develop clinical skills that will alert you when a dose is incorrect.

Hyperalimentation

Frequently, pharmacy technicians will be involved in the preparation of parenteral hyperalimentation solutions, also referred to as total parenteral nutrition (TPN) or just plain old "hyperal." These are complex intravenous infusions containing various nutrients, including vitamins, amino acids, dextrose, electrolytes, and trace elements. They will also frequently contain fat, insulin, and a variety of additional drugs. It is important for you to understand how to calculate hyperal solutions, even though most pharmacies today have computer programs that perform these functions.

Partial Hyperalimentation Formula *(for example only)*

500 ml of 8.5% amino acid injection
0.5 L of 70% dextrose injection
Sodium chloride 35 mEq
Calcium gluconate 7 mEq
Multivitamins 5 ml
Potassium chloride 30 mEq
Sodium phosphate 9 mM
Sodium acetate 45 mEq
Ranitidine 150 mg
Vitamin K 1000 mcg
Regular insulin 8 units

Questions: Determine the amount of each component source (below) required to prepare this hyperal order. Use ratio and proportion for each question, and cover the answers to see if you can calculate them on your own. (Don't peek!)

Component source	Volume needed	Answer
1-liter bottle of 8.5% amino acid injection	_____ L	0.5 liter
1000-ml bottle of 70% dextrose injection	_____ ml	500 ml
30-ml vial of sodium chloride (4 mEq/ml)	_____ ml	8.75 ml
10-ml vial of calcium gluconate (4.65 mEq/vial)	_____ ml	15 ml
10-ml vial of multivitamins	_____ vial	0.5 vial
10-ml vial of potassium chloride (2 mEq/ml)	_____ vial	1.5 vials
10-ml vial of sodium phosphate (3 mM/ml)	_____ ml	3 ml
20-ml vial of sodium acetate (2 mEq/ml)	_____ 1 vial + ml	1 vial + 2.5 ml
2-ml syringe of ranitidine (25 mg/ml)	_____ syringes	3 syringes
0.5-ml amp of vitamin K (2 mg/ml)	_____ amps	1 amp
10-ml vial of regular insulin (100 units/ml)	_____ ml	0.08 ml

PRACTICE

1. Without looking back, write the meaning of the following abbreviations.

   (a)   aa

   (b)   ad.

   (c)   q.s.

   (d)   D.T.D.

   (e)   M.

   (f)   ft.

2. How many grams of acetaminophen would be required to prepare 5,000 tablets of a narcotic analgesic if 1 tablet is to contain 10 mg of the narcotic and 325 mg of acetaminophen?

3. A cold capsule contains 30 mg of pseudoephedrine, 2 mg of brompheniramine, and 200 mg of ibuprofen. How many grams of each drug are required to make 100 of these cold capsules?

   (a)   Pseudoephedrine

   (b)   Brompheniramine

   (c)   Ibuprofen

4. If a diphenhydramine elixir contains 12.5 mg of diphenhydramine per tsp., how many grams would be required to prepare a pint of the elixir?

5. An antacid tablet contains 500 mg of calcium carbonate. How many kilograms of calcium carbonate are required to manufacture 10,000 bottles of the antacid tablets if there are 150 tablets per bottle? **This should keep you busy!**

6. From the following formula, calculate the number of grams of each ingredient required to prepare 2 kilograms of the ointment:

Precipitated sulfur	10 g
Salicylic acid	2 g
Hydrophilic ointment	88 g

(a)   Precipitated sulfur

(b)   Salicylic acid

(c)   Hydrophilic ointment

7. From the formula in Question 6 determine how many grams of each ingredient are required to prepare 60 grams of the ointment.

(a)   Precipitated sulfur

(b)   Salicylic acid

(c)   Hydrophilic ointment

8. How much of each ingredient would be required to prepare 45 grams of the following mixture? *(These are all solids to be weighed.)*

Camphor	0.3
Menthol	2
Talc	90
Zinc oxide qs 120	

(a)   Camphor

(b)   Menthol

(c)   Talc

(d)   Zinc oxide

9. From the formula in Question 8, determine how many grams of each ingredient are required to prepare 1 lb of the mixture.

(a)   Camphor

(b)   Menthol

(c)   Talc

(d)   Zinc oxide

10. From the following formula, determine how many milliliters of glycerin are required to prepare one pint of the syrup. *(These are all liquids.)*

Glycerin		90
Ipecac fluid extract		70
Syrup	qs	1000

11. From the formula in Question 10, determine how much ipecac fluid extract would be required to prepare 1 gallon of the syrup.

12. The following is an old capsule formula that a veterinarian likes to use:

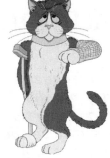

Hydralazine	15 mg
Reserpine	75 µg
Furosemide	20 mg

D.T.D. capsules #30

(a)   How many milligrams of reserpine are required to prepare this prescription?

(b)   How many grams of furosemide are required to fill this prescription?

(c)   What is the total weight in milligrams of the three drugs in one capsule?

(d)   What is the total weight in grams of the three drugs in all 30 capsules?

(e)   If the prescription had *"M. ft."* instead of *"D.T.D.,"* how many micrograms of hydralazine would be contained in one capsule?

▼▼▼▼▼ *The answers to all problems can be found in the answer key starting on page 160.* ▼▼▼▼▼

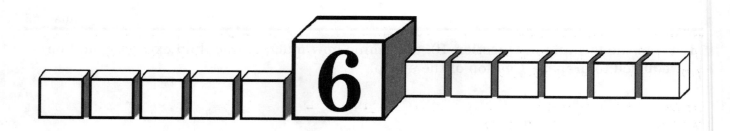

RECONSTITUTION OF DRY POWDERS

You will frequently have the opportunity to reconstitute or compound drugs that are in a dry powder form. These are usually drugs such as antibiotics, which lose their potency in a short period of time after being prepared in a liquid dosage form. Because they lose their potency so quickly, it is important not to reconstitute with water or other appropriate diluent until it is time to dispense.

Most oral preparations are formulated so that the "normal" dose will be contained in 1 teaspoonful of the solution. In this chapter, you will learn more about compounding these dry powder products.

OBJECTIVES

Upon mastery of Chapter 6 you will be able to:

Establish how much of a drug is contained in a vial or bottle.
Calculate the powder volume displacement of a reconstituted drug.
Solve problems related to dry powders.

This morning I prepared some good old fashioned oatmeal for breakfast. In preparing the oatmeal, I used 1 cup of dry oats and 2 cups of water. I assumed there would be about 3 cups of cooked oatmeal, but, to my surprise, there were approximately $2\frac{1}{4}$ cups. How in the world can you take 1 and add 2 and come up with approximately $2\frac{1}{4}$?

In this example, there are actually two things that contribute to the smaller than expected volume. First, there was some water evaporation from boiling. Second, the volume the "dry" oats displaced actually constricted and became much smaller when water was added. If you think about this, you will realize the dry oats have a lot of air between them, and you can actually compress the cup of oats to about $\frac{1}{3}$ cup by simply applying pressure. In this chapter, we will learn how to determine the volume a dry powder occupies in a reconstituted medicinal solution.

To establish the powder volume, simply subtract the volume of the diluent from the final volume of the solution.

In the oatmeal example, the diluent was the 2 cups of water, and our final product was the $2\frac{1}{4}$ cups of oatmeal.

$2\frac{1}{4}$ cups cooked oatmeal $-$ 2 cups water $= \frac{1}{4}$ cup

This means the *powder volume* of the dry oats was actually only $\frac{1}{4}$ cup.

 You will see various formulas for solving for powder volume, but, as I stated in the Preface, I cannot stand to memorize formulas. All you need to do is use common sense and subtract from your final volume the amount of water added and you will easily recognize the dry powder volume.

Reconstituting Drugs

Let's try a pharmacy-related problem.

Question: Based on what you have learned in previous chapters, how much tetracycline would be in a 150-ml bottle of tetracycline that says 250 mg/5 ml on the label?

Solution: By now, this should be an easy concept for you.
You can solve for the answer by simple ratio and proportion.

250 mg tetracycline/5 ml $=$?/150 ml

7,500 mg tetracycline $=$?

Question: When you prepare to reconstitute (i.e., add water) to the bottle of tetracycline in the previous question, you read on the label that you must add 117 ml of water to the bottle of prepackaged tetracycline powder. Based on the information given, what is the *powder volume* of the tetracycline in the bottle?

Solution: Take your final volume of 150 ml (this information is on the bottle) and simply subtract the volume of water that has been added (117 ml).

150 ml *final volume* $-$ 117 ml *water added* $=$ 33 ml *powder volume*

 There are two very important points I want you to remember. These are "no-brainers" that many people fail to understand. First, the amount of the drug in the bottle never changes. In the tetracycline example, there were 7,500 mg of tetracycline in the bottle. No matter whether you add 1 ml or 200 ml of water to the bottle, the amount of tetracycline remains constant; only the final volume changes. Second, the "powder volume" also remains the same. It will be 33 ml no matter what the final volume may be.

Question: In this tetracycline example, let's pretend you accidentally added 150 ml of water instead of 117 ml?

In the "real" world of pharmacy, it would be best to throw this bottle out and start over, but please bear with me for the sake of this example and consider you have messed up the last bottle of tetracycline in the universe!

How much tetracycline is in the bottle?   (answer: 7,500 mg)

What is the powder volume of the tetracycline?   (answer: 33 ml)

What is the final volume?   (answer: 183 ml)

Solution: 150 ml of water + 33 ml powder volume = 183 ml

Now put on your thinking cap!

How many milligrams of tetracycline are in a teaspoonful of the "messed-up" product?

Solution: 7,500 mg tetracycline/183 ml   =   ?/5 ml

                  205 mg tetracycline =   ?

How many milliliters of the "messed-up" product would you have to take to get the prescribed dose of 250 mg?

Solution: 7,500 mg tetracycline/183 ml   =   250 mg tetracycline/?

                  6.1 ml =   ?

(You could also have said 205 mg tetracycline/5 ml   =   250 mg/?)

PRACTICE

1. The label on a 200-ml bottle of ampicillin 125 mg/5 ml directs you to add 158 ml of water.

   (a) How much ampicillin is in the bottle?

   (b) What is the powder volume of the ampicillin in the bottle?

   (c) What would be the final volume if you accidentally added 178 ml of water?

   (d) How much ampicillin would be in 10 ml of the "messed-up" reconstitution in (c)?

   (e) How many milliliters of the "messed-up" ampicillin in (c) would be required to deliver a 250-mg dose?

2. The label on a 150-ml bottle of cefaclor 125 mg/5 ml directs you to add 111 ml of water.

   (a) How many milligrams of cefaclor are in the bottle?

   (b) What is the dry powder volume of cefaclor in the bottle?

Let's see how good you really are!

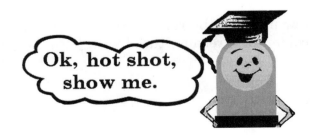

Ok, hot shot, show me.

(c)   If the physician wants you to prepare a cefaclor suspension to contain 100 mg/5 ml, how much additional water would you add?

(d)   Pretend you accidentally reconstituted the cefaclor bottle with 78 ml of water. How much cefaclor would be in a teaspoonful of this "incorrectly" reconstituted solution?

(e)   How many milliliters of the "messed-up" cefaclor in (d) would provide a 100-mg dose?

3. The label on a vial directs you to "add 7.8 ml of sterile water" to prepare a 10-ml "multidose" vial of a 100-mg/ml injection.

(a)   How many milliliters of the reconstituted solution for injection would provide a 300-mg dose?

(b)   How many grams of the drug are in one vial?

(c)   If a patient is to receive 250 mg q.i.d. x 10 d, how many multidose vials will be required?

(d)   What is the powder volume of the drug in this vial?

(e)   How much of the reconstituted solution would provide a 250-mg dose if you accidentally reconstituted with 9.8 ml of sterile water?

Here is a tough one. Good luck!

4. You are directed to reconstitute a vial of a drug. The label states that there are 10 million units of drug in the bottle, and, when reconstituted, you will have an injection containing 500,000 units/ml. **The drug has a dry powder volume = 7 ml.**

(a)   How many milliliters will provide a 2,500,000-unit dose?

(b)   How many total milliliters will be in a reconstituted bottle?

(c)   How much sterile water for injection should you add to correctly reconstitute this injection?

(d)   How many units would be in 1 ml of the injection if the vial was reconstituted with 20 ml of sterile water for injection?

(e)   In (d), how much of the incorrectly reconstituted injection would provide the 2,500,000-unit dose?

▼▼▼▼▼ *The answers to all problems can be found in the answer key starting on page 160.* ▼▼▼▼▼

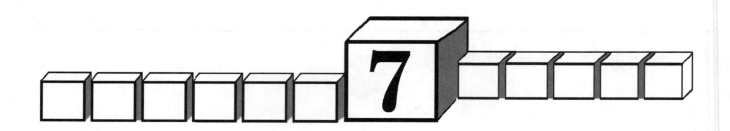

INTRAVENOUS FLOW RATES

*M*any pharmacy technicians work in the community/retail setting and have little or no exposure to intravenous (IV) solutions. Those of you working in hospitals and home healthcare have likely prepared numerous IV preparations. It is important for those in community practice to have an understanding of IVs because you never know when you might switch to a different area of practice where knowledge of IVs is essential.

I know five pharmacy technicians who have made big changes in their area of practice. The most frequent comment I hear from those technicians and others considering a career change from retail to hospital is, "I don't know anything about IVs." In fact, I know technicians who will not make a change based on that one factor. Preparing IVs is a skill you need to learn on the job or in a laboratory and is beyond the scope of this textbook.

In this chapter, I will familiarize you with "math" related issues concerning IV flow rates. In later chapters, we will discuss several other topics related to intravenous solutions. Again, I will not have you learn a bunch of "formulas." All the calculations in this chapter will be done by simple ratio and proportion.

OBJECTIVES

Upon mastery of Chapter 7 you will be able to:

Calculate the rate of delivery of IVs in milliliters per hour.
Convert milliliter flow rates to drops per minute.
Determine when an IV solution will run out based on flow rate.

As a pharmacy technician, you need to be aware of issues regarding flow rates, even though you will rarely determine them. Rates of delivery of IVs and other medications are usually determined by the physician in a medical order. The IV is then administered by the nurse. In many cases, pharmacists will also be involved.

Go with the Flow

So why do you need to know about this flow rate stuff? Because, based on flow rate calculations, you as a pharmacy technician will have a better understanding of how long certain IVs will last before needing to be resupplied.

More importantly, by being aware of appropriate flow rates for various drugs and IV solutions, you can play an important role in assuring that mistakes are not made. I know of two critical instances where pharmacy technicians played important roles in recognizing errors in rates of administration of drugs delivered by the intravenous route. I also recently saw a patient die because no one caught a flow rate error.

Now let's get to work and master flow rates.

*Large-volume parenteral solutions are usually administered to the patient either by allowing the solution to slowly drip by gravity flow into the patient's vein or through the use of electrical infusion pumps. Generally, the gravitational equipment will state the **drop factor** in drops per milliliter (gtt/ml). The majority of IV administration sets deliver 10, 12, 15, 20, or 60 gtt/ml. Sets with other volumes of delivery are also available, but are not as common. The electronic pumps can be set at various flow rates.*

Example: If an IV set is calibrated to deliver 20 gtt/ml, how many drops would deliver 60 ml of solution?

Many people use formulas for these questions, but I bet you can work them without memorizing some crazy formula you would probably forget 3 years from now!

Solution: Guess what? All you need to do is ratio and proportion, again!

20 gtt/1 ml = ?/60 ml

1,200 gtt = ?

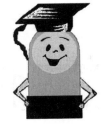

Are you still estimating your answers?

Example: Let's look at a question from the opposite direction. What would be the "calibration" in gtt/ml of an IV infusion set that delivers 90 milliliters with 1,350 drops?

Solution: Using ratio and proportion, simply say, "if there are 1,350 gtt in 90 ml, then there are **?** gtt in 1 ml."

$$1{,}350 \text{ gtt}/90 \text{ ml} \;=\; ?/1 \text{ ml}$$

$$15 \text{ gtt} \;=\; ?$$

The answer 15 gtt means the IV set is calibrated to deliver 15 gtt/ml.

Example: How many milliliters per minute would a patient receive if 200 ml of IV solution is being infused over a 2-hour period?

Solution: I like to change the hours to minutes whenever I am asked to provide a flow rate. This is especially helpful when the question asks for *ml/min* or *gtt/min.*

Step 1.   2 hours = 120 minutes

Step 2. $200 \text{ ml}/120 \text{ min} \;=\; ?/1 \text{ min}$

                   $1.67 \text{ ml} \;=\; ?$

Now let's "crank it up a notch"!

Try to work this example without looking at the solution.

Example: How many drops per minute would administer the IV solution in the above example if an IV set calibrated at 12 gtt/ml is used?

Solution: There are two ways to work this problem, and both are easy. The first solution uses the answer of 1.67 ml/min and converts it to gtt/min.

12 gtt/1 ml = ?/1.67 ml

20 gtt = ?

This means the 1.67 milliliters per minute is equivalent to 20 drops per minute.

The second solution converts the original volume of 200 ml in 2 hours to drops per minute. Both solutions require two steps each, so pick your favorite one.

Step 1.   12 gtt/1 ml = ?/200 ml

2,400 gtt = ?

Step 2.   2,400 gtt/120 min = ?/1 min

20 gtt = ?

Now it's your turn to try to put it all together. Remember these IV drip rate problems usually require several ratio and proportions, so be patient and organized.

Question: A physician writes a medication order for a liter of D5W to be administered to a patient over a 6-hour period. If the nurse uses an IV administration set that is calibrated at 10 gtt/ml, how many drops per minute should be delivered to the patient?

Solution 1:   Volume equals 1,000 ml delivered over 360 minutes (6 hours).

Step 1.   1,000 ml/360 min = ?/1 min

2.78 ml = ?

This means that 2.78 ml will be infused each minute.

Step 2.   10 gtt/1 ml = ?/2.78 ml

27.8 gtt = ?

This means the IV set will deliver 27.8 gtt per minute, which is the same volume as 2.78 ml. The 27.8 gtt would be rounded off to 28 gtt in the real world.

Solution 2:   **Step 1.**   10 gtt/1 ml = ?/1,000 ml

10,000 gtt = ?

This means the liter will have 10,000 drops when using the 10-gtt/ml delivery set.

Step 2.   10,000 gtt/360 min = ?/1 min

27.8 gtt = ?

PRACTICE

1. A physician orders 1,200 milliliters of normal saline to be infused in 8 hours.

   (a)   How many milliliters will be infused every hour?

   (b)   How many milliliters will be infused in 5 minutes?

   (c)   How many drops would be in the entire volume if an IV set calibrated at 15 gtt/ml is used?

   (d)   How many drops per minute must be infused using the 15-gtt/ml set to deliver the entire volume?

   (e)   If the solution contains 2 g of a drug, how many milligrams of the drug will the patient receive per hour?

2. A physician orders 500 milliliters of D5W to run for 8 hours.

   (a)   Calculate the flow rate in ml/min.

   (b)   Calculate the flow rate in gtt/min using an infusion set calibrated at 60 gtt/ml.

(c) If the nurse mistakenly set the flow rate at 2 ml/min, how many minutes would the solution run?

(d) What would the drip rate be in (c)?

(e) If the solution contains 2 mg of a drug, how many micrograms of the drug would be in 1 milliliter?

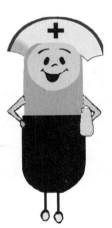

3. A patient receives 40 gtt/minute of an IV solution.

(a) How many milliliters per minute would the patient receive if the nurse is using an IV set calibrated at 15 gtt/ml?

(b) How many milliliters of fluid will the patient receive daily if the nurse uses the IV set in (a)?

(c) Based on your answer to (b), how many liter bags of IV fluid will have to be prepared for this patient for a 24-hour period?

(d) If this solution contains 1 gram of a medication per liter, how many milligrams of the drug will the patient receive per hour?

(e) Based on the information in (d), how many mcg of the drug will the patient receive per minute?

4. A physician orders a patient to receive 2 million units of ampicillin in a 1000-ml bag of an intravenous solution to be infused over 6 hours.

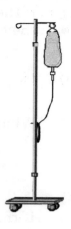

(a) How many milliliters of solution will the patient receive per hour?

(b) How many units of ampicillin will the patient receive per hour?

(c) How many units of ampicillin will the patient receive per minute?

(d) What is the flow rate in milliliters per minute?

(e) How many drops per hour would the patient receive if the nurse uses an IV set that delivers 12 gtt/ml?

(f) How many units of ampicillin would be in a single drop of solution if an IV set delivering 12 gtt/ml is used?

5. A patient is to receive 100 mg of a drug per hour in an IV solution for a period of 24 hours. The total daily IV volume is 2000 ml.

(a)   How many grams of the drug must the patient receive daily?

(b)   How many milliliters must the patient receive per hour to get the appropriate dose?

(c)   What is the flow rate in milliliters per minute?

(d)   What is the flow rate in drops per minute using a venoset calibrated at 15 gtt/ml?

(e)   How many milliliters of IV fluid will the patient receive in 5 hours?

(f)   How many milligrams of drug will the patient receive in 3.5 hours?

▼▼▼▼▼ *The answers to all problems can be found in the answer key starting on page 160.* ▼▼▼▼▼

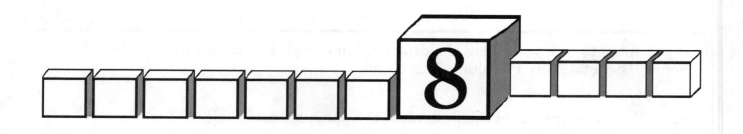

PERCENTAGE CALCULATIONS

*A*n area of study in pharmacy math that often gives practitioners a tough time is percentage calculations. You will frequently encounter percentages in everyday pharmacy practice, so it is important to have a solid understanding of this concept. Many pharmaceutical products from IV solutions to topicals are labeled in percents.

It has been my experience that pharmacy technicians and pharmacy students usually understand the concepts covered in the previous chapters, but fall apart when they hit percentage calculations. My goal in Chapter 8 is to make sure you have both a firm understanding of and an appreciation for percentages. I hope (in some perverted way) you will also have fun learning and applying the concepts in this chapter.

OBJECTIVES

Upon mastery of Chapter 8 you will be able to:

Define the concept of percent strength.
Convert among percents, fractions, decimals, and ratios.
Solve for the quantity of a drug in a compound given its percent strength.
Understand the different types of percents.
Differentiate between percent and milligram percent.
Relate parts per million to percent strength.
Properly write ratio strengths.

I know you already have been exposed to the concept of percent for many years, but do you really understand what it means? My experience is that most people can solve basic problems related to percents, but in reality they are just going through the math procedures without completely grasping what is really going on. So if I appear to be "spoon-feeding" you in this chapter, you are very perceptive because I am.

Now let's see what you know about basic percents and then advance to a higher level. Oh yeah, I thought you might like to know that the math in this chapter still does not go beyond basic ratio and proportion. Furthermore, there are no formulas to memorize for at least another chapter, so I am keeping my promises as much as possible.

Now let's go have fun and take the fear out of percent calculations.

Example: If you took a 100-question history final examination and got 94 questions correct, what would be your score on the exam?
Please don't tell me the answer is "an A"!

Solution: I bet you correctly figured this out to be 94%, so you get your A. In this example, you simply applied the definition of **percent (%),** which is *parts per hundred,* and then solved the question. In other words, you stated:

*94 parts per 100 **or** 94 questions per 100 questions equals 94%*

Always remember that percent means "parts per hundred,"
and you will easily understand the rest of Chapter 8.

Another method for solving percent problems is by dividing the number of correct answers by the *total* number of questions: $\frac{94}{100} = 0.94$.

Wait a minute. How can 0.94 be 94%? If you do not understand how this can be, then please go back to the definition of *percents*. If *percent* is defined as *parts per hundred*, the answer 0.94 means what? It means $\frac{94}{100}$ or 94 parts/100 parts. Now take the 0.94 and move the decimal 2 places to the right and add a percent sign (%). This means 0.94 is exactly the same as $\frac{94}{100}$, which is exactly the same as saying 94%, which is exactly the same as what ratio? The answer is exactly 94:100.

I know, I know, it is a whole lot simpler to just say you got an A!

Example: If you are a cattle rancher in South America and have 100 steers and 65 die from cholera, what percent of your steers died?

Solution: Hopefully you said 65% without a whole lot of effort. Again, we can restate these numbers in many ways. We can say 65 steers out of 100 steers **or** 0.65 **or** 65 parts out of 100 parts **or** $\frac{65}{100}$ **or** 65% **or** 65:100. These terms all mean the same thing. Oh, by the way, what ratio of steers is still alive? The answer is 35:100, which again is the same as $\frac{35}{100}$, 0.35, and 35%.

The percents will always add up to 100%. In this case 35% + 65% = 100%.

Hopefully you are still awake and you understand what we have covered so far. If you have not grasped the concepts in the first two examples, do not proceed until you are very comfortable with these basic concepts of percents. **It may be time to ask your instructor for help if this is getting a little bit confusing.** But if you are ready, then let's crank-it-up a notch using the same examples with a few minor changes to see if you are as smart as you think you are. I bet you are actually smarter.

Example: If you took a 135-question history final examination and got 94 questions correct, what would your score on the exam be (other than bad)?

Solution: You didn't do well on this exam, especially if 70% was passing. Did you calculate your score on this test to be 69.6%? If so, you are well on the way to mastering this topic, but did you think about this question as *parts per hundred,* or did you just divide 94 by 135? Right now the latter solution works, but I need you to start thinking beyond just dividing numbers in order to assure you understand later. Ways to answer this question include:

$$\frac{94}{135} = 0.696 \rightarrow 69.6\%$$

OR

94 questions/135 questions = ?/100 questions

Based on years of experience, I would bet you used the first method. I prefer that you use the second because it defines the process better. The second choice is no more difficult. It is just plain old-fashioned ratio and proportion. When solving this problem, did you actually think about the percent being the number of questions you got right out of 100 instead of 135?

You probably did not because most people rarely think of percents on this level. Again, it will be easier for you in the long run if you solve percents as *parts per hundred*. With this in mind, the answer 69.6% actually means that you averaged 69.6 questions right out of 100. Pretty cool, huh! Let me give you an example of how this could work in reverse.

Example: If you score 69.6% on a history final examination, how many questions did you get right out of 135 questions?

Solution: If 69.6% means 69.6 parts per 100, then _____ parts would be right in 135.

$$\frac{69.6}{100} = \frac{?}{135}$$

Some people multiply 135 times 0.696 to get 94, but do they understand what is happening in this calculation? Again, I prefer the ratio method.

Now you try one based on a previous example. Please work it by ratio and proportion and parts per hundred.

Question: If you are a cattle rancher in South America and have 82 steers and 65 die from cholera, what percent of your steers lived?

Solution: If you had 82 steers and lost 65, then only 17 steers survived.

17 steers/82 *total* steers = ?/100 steers

20.7 steers = **?**

20.7 out of 100 = **20.7% survived**

Question: In the previous question, what percent of the steers died?

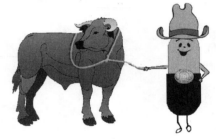

Solution: 100% − 20.7% = **79.3% died.**
This can also be solved by ratio and proportion:

$$\frac{65}{82} = \frac{?}{100}$$

79.3 = ? $(\frac{73.9}{100} = 79.3\%)$

Question: If another farmer lost 39% of his cattle to cholera, how many steers did he have to start with if 325 steers died?

Solution: This one is a little tougher, but just think it out. What does 39% mean? It means that 39 steers died out of every 100 steers. Now set up the ratio and proportion.   39 steers died/100 steers = 325 steers died/?

833 total steers = ? (i.e., the entire herd)

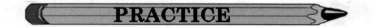

PRACTICE

1. Find the equivalent percent, fraction, decimal, and ratio for the following:

	Percent	Fraction	Decimal	Ratio
(a)	_____	$\frac{3}{16}$	_____	_____
(b)	_____	$\frac{2}{11}$	_____	_____
(c)	18%	_____	_____	_____
(d)	3.5%	_____	_____	_____
(e)	_____	_____	0.61	_____
(f)	_____	_____	0.08	_____
(g)	_____	_____	_____	1:125
(h)	_____	_____	_____	35:400

2. Yesterday I bought a gallon of skim milk and I need your help:

    (a)   What percent of the milk I bought yesterday is a 12-fluid ounce glassful?

    (b)   If my wife Patricia drank a pint of the milk, what percent did she drink?

OK, so you think you are good. Try this one!

(c)   If Patricia drank a pint, my son Billy drank a quart, my daughters Kim and Angela *each* drank 6 ounces, and my baby Abby drank 120 ml, what percent of the gallon of milk did they drink?

(d)   What percent of the milk remains for me and the dogs and cats after my family has consumed the volumes in (c)?

3. Last week I took my family trout fishing and all *six* of us caught the limit of five trout apiece. (We fudged a little with the infant's limit!)

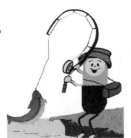

(a)   What percent of the trout did each member of my family catch?

(b)   What percent of the trout did my four children catch?

(c)   If the total weight of all the trout was 22.5 pounds, how many kilograms did all the trout weigh?

(d)   Based on your answer to (c), what percent of the total weight did our largest trout weigh if it weighed 950 grams?

(e)   My family had 18 trout get away after hooking them. Considering the number we caught and those that escaped to fight another day, what percent did we lose?

4. If you ate a 1-lb steak and it had a 25% fat content, how many grams of fat did you consume?

5. If you ate 14 ounces of pork chops and they contained 4 ounces of fat, what percent of the pork chops was fat?

6. My wife Patricia runs marathons for fun. (I'm not really sure how running 26.2 miles can be fun, but she loves it!) She says the toughest part of the race is when she gets to the "wall" which for her is around mile number 21. What percent of a 26.2-mile marathon has she completed when she hits the wall?

7. I noticed on a 448-gram can of Great Northern beans that the can contains 2% fat, 28 g protein, 2 g sodium, 18 g fiber, and 68 g carbohydrate.

(a) What is the percent protein in the beans?

(b) How many grams of fat are in a can?

(c) What percent of the can is *not* carbohydrate?

▼▼▼▼▼ *The answers to all problems can be found in the answer key starting on page 160.* ▼▼▼▼▼

I bet you are wondering what all this has to do with pharmacy. Actually, we will now start relating the concepts you have (hopefully) learned to your practice setting.
I want you to remember that the process doesn't change, just the context we will be working in. So goodbye to fat grams, marathons, trout fishing, and cholera-infested steers, and hello to IV solutions, antifungals, glaucoma medications, and potassium supplements.

Percentage Preparations

In pharmacy practice, you will encounter three types of percentage preparations, which are determined by the physical nature of the components in a particular product. Percentage concentrations are expressed as follows:

Percent weight-in-weight (w/w) or (wt/wt)

Percent volume-in-volume (v/v) or (vol/vol)

Percent weight-in-volume (w/v) or (wt/vol)

Percent Weight-in-Weight (w/w) or (wt/wt)

*This percent expresses the number of parts of a constituent in 100 parts of a preparation. Are you wondering what a **part** is? It can actually be just about anything. For example, to prepare rice you could say add 1 part rice to 2 parts water. This could mean 1 cup rice to 2 cups water, or it could also mean 1 handful of rice to 2 handfuls of water. Just remember, this parts lingo is really just talking about a ratio of one quantity to another. In the case of the rice, we want to always use twice as much water as rice which is the same as saying "2 parts to 1 part" or "2:1."*

With weight-in-weight percents, the parts could be in grams, grains, pounds, ounces, kilograms, or any other weight. This type of percent is used for measuring the weight of a substance in the total weight of a product. The final product is usually a solid or semisolid. Examples of these products are powders, ointments, and creams. This may be a little bit confusing, so let's look at a few examples.

Example: What would be the weight of zinc oxide (ZnO) in 120 grams of 10% zinc oxide ointment?

Solution: Because an *ointment* is a semisolid, it is normally **weighed,** and we usually express the weight in grams even though other units of weight may be used. Zinc oxide is the "active" ingredient in the zinc oxide ointment. Zinc oxide is a solid powder, so it too is weighed. This problem is no different from previous examples. Just think of the grams as steers or trout, and you will do just fine. I know you are going to be tempted to just multiply 10% or 0.1 times 120 g to get the answer (and that is a correct way of doing it), but I will again work it by ratio and proportion to make sure you understand the total process. Having a 10% zinc oxide ointment means there are 10 grams of zinc oxide in 100 grams of the final ointment. So by ratio and proportion we can solve the problem in the following manner:

10 g **zinc oxide**/100 g **ointment** = ?/120 g **ointment**

12 g **zinc oxide** = ?

Example: How many grams of zinc oxide would be in 1 lb of 5% zinc oxide ointment?

Solution: This example is solved in the same manner as the previous one, but with one exception. When solving weight-in-weight problems, the *units must always be the same*. So you will need to convert the "pound" to "grams."

5 g **zinc oxide**/100 g **ointment** = ?/1 lb **ointment**

5 g **zinc oxide**/100 g **ointment** = ?/454 g **ointment**

22.7 g **zinc oxide** = ?

To check your answer, take the amount of zinc oxide (22.7 g) and divide it by the total weight (454 g)
22.7/454 = 0.05 = 5/100 = 5% zinc oxide

NOW YOU TRY TO ANSWER A COUPLE OF QUESTIONS.

Question: What would be the percent strength of a zinc oxide ointment if you prepared 90 grams of an ointment that contained 5 grams of zinc oxide?

Solution: If the *final* product weighs 90 grams and it contains 5 grams of zinc oxide, then to solve for the percent strength you set up a ratio and proportion to see how much zinc oxide would be in 100 g of ointment.

5 g **zinc oxide**/90 g **ointment** = ?/100 g **ointment**

5.56 g **zinc oxide** = ?

This means there are 5.56 g ZnO per 100 g of ointment, i.e., **5.56%**

To check your answer, just multiply 5.56% (0.556) times 90 g to get 5 g, which is the amount of zinc oxide you used to make the ointment.

Now that you think you are the master of percents, try this tricky question.

Question: What would be the percent strength of a zinc oxide ointment if you *added* 90 grams of an ointment base to 5 grams of zinc oxide?

OOPS! Did I just ask you this question?

Solution: Contrary to what you might think, this is **not similar** to the previous question. In the other question, I said the 90 g of ointment *contained* the 5 g of zinc oxide. In this question I said you *added* 5 grams of zinc oxide *to* 90 grams of an ointment base. In the first question, the final weight was 90 grams, but in this one the final weight would be 95 grams.

5 g **zinc oxide**/95 g **ointment** = ?/100 g **ointment**

5.26 g **zinc oxide** = ?

5.26/100 = 5.26%

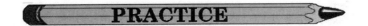

PRACTICE

8. If you were to prepare 150 g of a coal tar ointment containing 12 g of coal tar,

(a)   What is the percent strength of coal tar in the ointment?

(b)   What would be the percent strength of coal tar in 1 mg of ointment?

9. If you prepare a powder that contains 2 mg of a drug in every gram of powder,

(a)   How much of the drug would be in 120 grams of the powder?

(b)   What is the percent strength of the drug in the powder?

10. If you were to prepare a topical cream containing 3% hydrocortisone,

(a)   How many grams of hydrocortisone would be required to prepare 1 pound of the topical cream?

(b)   How many milligrams of hydrocortisone would be in 1 g of the cream?

11. If 25 grams of Efudex® Cream contains 5% fluorouracil,

   (a)   How many milligrams of fluorouracil are in the cream?

   (b)   What would be the new percent strength if you *added* 2 g of fluorouracil to the Efudex Cream?

12. From the following formula: Hydrocortisone   1.5 g
                                                       Vioform powder   0.5 g
                                                       Cream base   ad   60 g

   (a)   What is the percent strength of hydrocortisone in this cream?

   (b)   How much cream base is required to prepare this prescription?

   (c)   How much Vioform® powder would be required to prepare 10 ounces of this cream?

13. From the following formula: Phenobarbital Na   60 mg
                                                          Aminophylline   200 mg
                                                          Carbowax base   1.8 g

   (a)   This formula is for one suppository; how many grams of aminophylline are required to prepare 60 suppositories?

   (b)   How much would the 60 suppositories weigh?

   (c)   What is the percent strength of phenobarbital in 60 suppositories?

14. From the following formula:

Benzocaine	1:1000
Precipitated sulfur	10%
Zinc oxide paste	ad 120 g

(a)   How many milligrams of benzocaine are in this prescription?

(b)   How many grams of precipitated sulfur would be required to prepare a kilogram of this product?

15. From the following formula:

Magnesium oxide	2 parts
Sodium bicarbonate	5 parts
Calcium carbonate	7 parts

(a)   How many grams of calcium carbonate are required to prepare 2 pounds of this powder?

(b)   What is the percent strength of sodium bicarbonate in the powder?

(c)   What is the ratio strength of magnesium oxide in the powder?

▼▼▼▼▼ *The answers to all problems can be found in the answer key starting on page 160.* ▼▼▼▼▼

Percent Volume-in-Volume (v/v) or (vol/vol)

A second type of percent is percent volume-in-volume. You will not see this type of percent very often, but you still need to have a working knowledge of such problems. Fortunately, percent (v/v) problems are worked in a similar manner as percent (w/w) problems. In the previous section, we discussed weight-in-weight percents where the active constituent (the drug) was weighed, and the final product was a solid and also weighed.

The percent volume-in-volume compounds are solution or liquid preparations, and the active constituents are also solutions or liquids. In most cases, we will measure the volumes of the final product and the constituents in milliliters. These types of problems can also be worked with other units of volume (i.e., pints, fluid ounces, quarts), but please do not forget that all units must be the same, just as we saw in the weight-in-weight problems.

Example: What would be the percent strength (v/v) of a pint of a solution that contains 1 fluid ounce of liquefied phenol?

Solution: Just as you did with the percent (w/w) problems, simply get everything into the same units and solve for parts per 100 to get the percent. In this example, a pint equals 480 ml and a fluid ounce contains 30 ml.

30 ml **liquefied phenol**/480 ml **solution** = ?/100 ml **solution**

6.25 ml **liquefied phenol** = ?

Every 100 ml of the solution contains 6.25 ml of liquefied phenol. 6.25 ml/100 ml = 6.25% (v/v)

You may have also said 30/480 = 0.0625 = 6.25%, but I still want you to work these problems by ratio and proportion.

Do you see an easier way to work this example? You could have said that a pint has 16 fluid ounces, and it contains 1 fluid ounce of liquefied phenol.

1 fl.ounce/16 fl.ounces = ?/100 fl.ounces

6.25 fl.ounces = ?

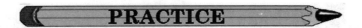

PRACTICE

16. A mouthwash contains 0.35% (v/v) of a mint flavoring.

   (a)   How many milliliters of flavoring are in a quart of mouthwash?

   (b)   If you have a gallon of this mouthwash, what would be the percent strength (v/v) of mint flavoring in 1 milliliter of mouthwash?

17. Six fluid ounces of a lotion contain 16 ml of resorcinol monoacetate.

   (a)   What is the percent strength of resorcinol monoacetate in this lotion?

   (b)   How many milliliters of resorcinol monoacetate would be required to prepare 5 liters of the lotion?

18. You have 1 pint of menthyl salicylate available.

(a)   How many gallons of a 6% menthyl salicylate lotion can be prepared?

(b)   How many milliliters of menthyl salicylate would be needed to prepare a pint of 6% menthyl salicylate lotion?

19. If verigreen spirits contains 5% verigreen oil, how many milliliters of the spirits can be prepared from a tablespoonful of verigreen oil?

20. If dynamint spirits contains 1:15 dynamint oil, how many milliliters of the spirits can be prepared from $\frac{1}{2}$ pint of dynamint oil?

▼▼▼▼▼ *The answers to all problems can be found in the answer key starting on page 160.* ▼▼▼▼▼

Percent Weight-in-Volume (w/v) or (wt/vol)

Last, but not least, is percent weight-in-volume, a percent you will frequently work with in most practice settings. As with the volume-in-volume percent problems, the final product in weight-in-volume percent is a solution or liquid preparation. The big difference is that the constituent or drug is measured by weight.

By now you have probably noticed a trend. In the abbreviations (w/w, v/v, and w/v), the denominator tells you if the final product is a solid or a liquid (i.e., measured by weight or volume), and the numerator gives you the same information about the constituent or drug. Unfortunately, you will rarely see these abbreviations next to a percent sign in the real world of medicine and pharmacy.

*You will eventually learn from experience how to recognize the different types of percents. In percent volume-in-volume (v/v) solutions, you may recall, the units could vary as long as they were the same kind of units. You could have pints per pints, milliliters per milliliters, quarts per quarts. In the percent weight-in-weight (w/w) preparations, the units could also vary but had to be the same kind of units. You could have g/g, kg/kg, lb/lb, gr/gr, etc. This is **not** the case with percent weight-in-volume. With % (w/v), the numerator or constituent is measured in grams only, and the denominator or final solution is measured in milliliters only. An example of this would be a solution of 10% potassium chloride. The 10% here means 10 grams KCl/100 milliliters solution.*

Example: What would be the percent (w/v) of a solution of potassium chloride that contains 24 grams of potassium chloride in 4 fluid ounces?

Solution: Do not forget to **always** solve these problems with *grams* of constituent over *100 milliliters* of final solution. In this example, we have 24 g/4 fl. oz. This needs to be changed to 24 **g**/120 **ml**.

24 **g KCl**/120 **ml solution** = ?/100 **ml solution**

20 **g KCl** = ?

20 g/100 ml = 20% (w/v)

Example: How many grams of potassium chloride would be in a pint of 10% KCl?

Solution: Change the pint to 480 milliliters. Ten percent means: 10 g KCl/100 ml.

10 **g KCl**/100 **ml solution** = ?/480 **ml solution**

48 **g KCl** = ?

In other words, if there are 10 g of KCl in 100 ml, then there must be 48 g of KCl in 480 ml of 10% solution.

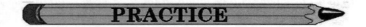

PRACTICE

21. You have a liter bag of normal saline (NS) that is 0.9% sodium chloride.

(a) How many grams of sodium chloride are contained in the bag?

(b) If a patient receives 200 ml of the NS every hour, how many milligrams of sodium chloride will he receive in 3 hours?

22. A $\frac{1}{2}$ liter IV solution contains 37.5 grams of sodium bicarbonate.

(a) What is the percent strength of sodium bicarbonate in the solution?

(b) How many milligrams of sodium bicarbonate are in 100 ml of solution?

(c) What is the percent sodium bicarbonate in 5 ml of the IV solution?

23. You have on hand 85 grams of iodine.

    (a)   What would be the percent strength of a gallon of iodine tincture compounded with the 85 grams?

    (b)   How many milliliters of 3% iodine tincture can be made from the amount of iodine on hand?

    (c)   How much of a 1:100 iodine tincture can be made from the amount of iodine on hand?   The 1:100 ratio means 1 g:100 ml.

Hint

24. Adenosine phosphate is available in 10-ml vials that contain 25 mg/ml.

    (a)   How many grams of adenosine phosphate are in a vial?

    (b)   What is the percent strength of adenosine phosphate?

    (c)   How many milliliters of adenosine phosphate would provide a 0.035-g dose?

25. Pilocarpine is available as a 0.5% solution.

    (a)   How many milligrams of pilocarpine are required to prepare 15 ml of the pilocarpine solution?

    (b)   If the dropper bottle delivers 18 drops of 5% pilocarpine solution in each milliliter, how many drops are in a 15-ml bottle of pilocarpine?

    (c)   Based on your answers to a and b, how many micrograms of pilocarpine are contained in 1 drop of the solution?

26. If 50 milligrams of nitroglycerin are in a liter of IV fluid:

(a) What is the percent strength of nitroglycerin?

(b) How many milliliters of the solution would deliver a 200-mcg dose?

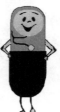

27. If a physician ordered a 15-mg "test dose" of a drug for a patient, how many milliliters of a 5% solution would be used to provide the dose?

▼▼▼▼▼ *The answers to all problems can be found in the answer key starting on page 160.* ▼▼▼▼▼

Milligram Percents (mg%)

If you are working in an institutional environment, you will sometimes see another type of percent referred to as a milligram percent (mg%). These milligram percents are not routinely used for dosing, but they are frequently used in reporting various clinical laboratory test results. They are used to report various chemicals that are present in the body in small quantities. Several examples are cholesterol, glucose, creatinine, and even some drugs.

In the last section you learned about weight-in-volume percents, which were measured as g/100 ml. The only difference with milligram percent problems is that the numerator is in milligrams instead of grams. Also, instead of seeing the 100 ml in the denominator, you will see the letters dL, which stand for a "deciliter" which is the same as 1/10 of a liter, which is the same as 100 ml.

So we are back to where we started!

Example: If a patient's serum glucose is reported as 165 mg/dL, express this as a mg%.

Solution: Remember that a deciliter (dL) equals 100 ml.

165 mg/dL = 165 mg/100 ml = *165 mg%*

Example: Express 165 mg% as a normal weight-in-volume percent.

Solution: If 165 mg equal 0.165 g, then you could say the following:

165 mg% = 165 mg/100 ml = 0.165 g/100 ml = *0.165%*

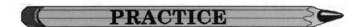

28. In most states, you would be considered legally drunk if you have a blood alcohol level of 200 mg/dL. Express this as a normal percent (w/v).

29. A patient has a serum creatinine of 0.15% (w/v). Express this as a mg%.

30. If a patient has a serum cholesterol level of 95 mg%, how many micrograms of cholesterol would be in 1 milliliter of serum?

▼▼▼▼▼ *The answers to all problems can be found in the answer key starting on page 160.* ▼▼▼▼▼

Parts Per Million (ppm)

As you saw in the last section, mg% is used to measure very small quantities. It is easier and safer to write 5 mg% rather than 0.005%. In this section, we will see a term that is used for even more dilute solutions than mg%. The term is parts per million (ppm). Probably the most common example of a substance measured in ppm is the fluoride in your drinking water. If your drinking water contains 2 ppm, this indicates there are 2 grams of fluoride in every "million" milliliters of water. This can also be written as a ratio: 2:1,000,000. As you can see, 2 ppm is less difficult to write than 0.0002%. The term ppm can also be used for weight-in-weight and volume-in-volume problems.

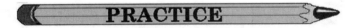

31. An antifungal is available in dry fish feed in a concentration of 8 ppm.

    (a)   Express this concentration as a ratio (reduce to lowest terms).

    (b)   Express this concentration as a percent (w/w).

    (c)   How many grams of antifungal would be in a kg of the feed?

32. How many grams of sodium fluoride would be required to prepare 1,000 gallons of a 1-ppm supply of fluoridated drinking water?

33. Express 0.00005% (w/v) in parts per million.

34. In Question 33, how many micrograms would be in a liter of solution?

Writing Ratio Strengths

Till now I have been letting you get away with writing ratios any way you wanted to because I wanted you to understand the basic concepts behind percents, fractions, and ratios. Now it is time for you to learn the proper format for writing ratios. This is a very simple process that once again uses ratio and proportion.

To write ratios properly, you should always have a 1 to the left of the colon. In other words, 5:25 would be incorrect. The correct way of writing this would be 1:5. In this example, we just divided both sides by 5 and reduced to lowest terms. But what would you do if the ratio was 5:13? To set this up correctly, just plug your numbers into another ratio and proportion using a 1 above the ?. By doing this, the 1 will represent the number to the left of the colon, and the number you get for the ? will represent the number to the right of the colon. This is how it will look:

$$\frac{5}{13} = \frac{?}{1} \qquad (or \quad 5{:}13 \quad equals \quad 1{:}?\,)$$

$$2.6 = ?$$

The ratio $\frac{5}{13}$ or 5:13 now becomes **1:2.6**.

To check your answer, divide both fractions and you will get the same decimal answer (5 divided by 13 equals 0.3846) and (1 divided by 2.6 equals 0.3846).

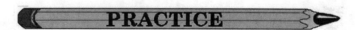

PRACTICE

35. Convert the following numbers to correctly written ratios:

(a)	2/7	(d)	0.125	(g)	2:23
(b)	17/510	(e)	0.08	(h)	23:300
(c)	33/135	(f)	0.45	(i)	48:200

▼▼▼▼▼ *The answers to all problems can be found in the answer key starting on page 160.* ▼▼▼▼▼

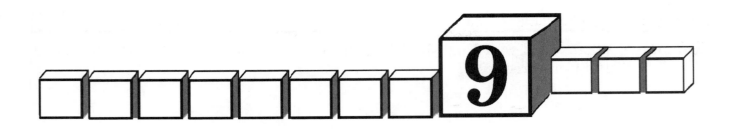

CONCENTRATIONS AND DILUTIONS

Please *do not continue until you have mastered Chapters 1 through 8. This chapter is based on your having a strong understanding of previous information, especially information related to ratios and percentages.*

*T*here will be times when you have to **compound** by reducing the strength of a **concentrated** (stock) product to a lower strength. This procedure is known as a **dilution.** Examples of dilutions are preparing a 5% IV solution from a 10% solution or preparing a 2% ointment by mixing 1% and 3% ointments.

In Chapter 9, I will teach you how to handle dilutions with as little pain as possible. Because of the uniqueness of dilutions, I have to veer a little from the ratio and proportion technique. In addition, I have to use a formula. I hate to have to do this, but hopefully you will forgive me once you become a dilution master!

OBJECTIVES

Upon mastery of Chapter 9 you will be able to:

Solve for the average percent of a mixture using alligation medial.
Determine the amount of a stock solution required to prepare a dilution.
Perform dilutions of liquid, semisolid, and solid dosage forms.
Explain how to determine mixture proportions using alligation alternate.
Calculate volumes and weights using specific gravity.

I would confidently bet that you have solved for the **average** of something during your tenure on earth! One thing that comes to mind are your grades in school. Now I am going to assume you are pretty bright, because you are already in Chapter 9 of this book. As an example, why don't we figure out your average in an English course.

Example: What would your English average have been if you had scored 80%, 90%, and 100% on three tests?

Solution: Hopefully, you added the numbers and divided by 3.

Step 1. $80 + 90 + 100 = 270$

Step 2. $270 \div 3 = $ **90%** (your average score)

Now you try solving several problems for the average.

Question: What would be the average weight of a steak if you bought four steaks that weighed $\frac{3}{4}$ pound, $\frac{1}{2}$ pound, $2\frac{1}{2}$ pounds, and 20 ounces?

Solution:
1

There are two ways to solve this question, and both require that all units be equal. In Solution 1, let's convert everything to pounds:

$$\tfrac{3}{4} \text{ lb} + \tfrac{1}{2} \text{ lb} + 2\tfrac{1}{2} \text{ lb} + 1\tfrac{1}{4} \text{ lb} = 5 \text{ lb}$$

Convert 20 ounces to pounds by saying: 16 oz/1 lb $=$ 20 oz/?

                                                       $1\frac{1}{4}$ lb $=$?

$5 \text{ lb} \div 4 \text{ steaks} = $ an average of $1\frac{1}{4}$ lb per steak

As a ratio and proportion, you would say, "If 4 steaks weigh 5 pounds, then 1 steak would weigh (?) pounds.
4 steaks/5 lb $=$ 1 steak/?
               $1\frac{1}{4}$ lb $=$?

Solution:
2

For this second solution, I again convert the weight of each steak to the same units. This time, I convert the pounds to ounces. Again, all I need to do is simple ratio and proportion.

Example: 1 lb/16 oz $= \frac{3}{4}$ lb/?
                12 oz $=$?

Now add all the ounces and divide by 4 steaks.
$12 \text{ oz} + 8 \text{ oz} + 40 \text{ oz} + 20 \text{ oz} = 80 \text{ oz}$
$80 \text{ oz} \div 4 \text{ steaks} = $ *20 oz per steak (same as $1\frac{1}{4}$ lb per steak)*

Question: My family has three cars (one doesn't run) that have varying fuel capacities. My wife's car holds 23.5 gallons of gasoline, my car holds 62 quarts, and the car that doesn't run holds 96 pints. What is the average fuel capacity?

Solution: Again, you need to convert to one unit. For this example, let's convert to quarts. Our answer will be the same if we convert to pints or gallons.

4 qt/1 gal = ?/23.5 gal   ? = 94 qt

2 pt/1 qt   = 96 pt/?   ? = 48 qt

Now add the quantities and divide by 3.

62 + 94 + 48 = 204 quarts (total for all three cars)

204 ÷ 3 = 68 quarts *(the average fuel capacity)*

Alligation Medial

Instead of an explanation, let's look at an example.

Example: Assume you move into a new seven-room home and decide to put telephones in every room except the two bathrooms. What would be the average cost of a telephone if you paid $32 for the family room phone, $48 for the kitchen phone, and $22 each for the three bedroom phones?

Solution: The hard way to work this is: $32 + $48 + $22 + $22 + $22 = $146

$146 ÷ 5 = *$29.20 per phone*

There is an easier way. Did you think of it?

1 phone	×	$32	= $32
1 phone	×	$48	= $48
+ 3 phones	×	$22	= $66
5 phones			**$146**

5 phones/$146 = 1 phone/? **or** $146/5 phones = $29.20 = cost of 1 phone

Guess what? This second solution is alligation medial, so you already know this techique! Now let's go apply it to the world of pharmacy practice.

PRACTICE

1. What is the average number of prescriptions that can be filled daily by the pharmacy technicians at a large city hospital if 12 technicians can each fill 100 prescriptions each day, 20 can each fill 125 prescriptions, 23 can each fill 150 prescriptions, and eight can fill 175 prescriptions?

2. What is the percent alcohol in a mixture of 2 liters of 20% alcohol, 1 liter of 50% alcohol, and 750 ml of 80% alcohol?

3. What is the percent concentration of potassium chloride in a mixture of 1 pint of 10% KCl, 3 quarts of 5% KCl, and 1 gallon of 20% KCl?

4. What would be the final percent strength of potassium chloride if you added 1 quart of water to the mixture in Question 3?

5. What would be the final percent of benzalkonium chloride in a mixture of 1 pint of 2% benzalkonium chloride and a liter of 6% benzalkonium chloride?

6. What would be the final percent concentration of benzalkonium chloride if you added $\frac{1}{2}$ liter of a 1:500 benzalkonium chloride solution to the mixture in Question 5?

 I highly recommend converting ratios to percents before working any of these *dilution* problems.

Now I bet I can trick you!

7. What is the percent strength of alcohol in a mixture of a liter of 95% alcohol, a quart of 70% alcohol, and a pint of 17% benzalkonium chloride?

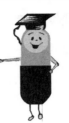

TIP: **Benzalkonium chloride is 0% alcohol.**

8. What is the percent strength of ichthammol in a mixture of 100 grams *each* of ichthammol ointments containing 5%, 15%, and 20%?

9. What would be the ratio strength of ichthammol in the ointment in Question 8 if you added 100 grams of pure ichthammol? **(For the purposes of this question, consider "pure" ichthammol to be 100%.)**

10. What would be the percent strength of a mixture of 1 lb of a 1:50 sulfur powder and 1 kilogram of a 1:20 sulfur powder?

▼▼▼▼ *The answers to all problems can be found in the answer key starting on page 160.* ▼▼▼▼

**Are you still estimating your answers?
If not, shame on you!**

Stock Solutions and Dilutions

Stock solutions are "concentrated" or "potent" solutions of medicinal substances that are frequently used to compound "weaker" solutions for human use. These stock solutions are very convenient because a pharmacist or pharmacy technician can prepare very large volumes of a product from small quantities of the stock solution.

You have probably used a form of a stock solution on several occasions in your own home. Examples I can think of at my home are insecticides, hardwood floor cleaners, hummingbird food, weed killer, and plant fertilizer. All of these products are in small bottles of concentrate that require dilution with water. Such products are stock solutions and would be dangerous to use without diluting. The advantage of the stock solution is that it saves you tons of space. In this section, we will learn how to prepare dilutions using stock solutions and other concentrates.

PLEASE NOTE: *Dilutions cannot be worked by simple ratio and proportion because there is an inverse relationship occurring and your answer will be way off base! Always, always, always estimate your answers, especially when you are working dilution problems.*

Now let's have some fun diluting!

The formula I like best for solving dilutions is : **(OV) (O%) = (NV) (N%)**

I know this looks pretty complicated, but it is a very easy formula to remember. The abbreviations stand for the following:

OV stands for *Old Volume*   *(This is the volume we are starting with.)*

O% stands for *Old %*   *(This is the percent concentration of the Old Volume.)*

NV stands for *New Volume*   *(This is the "new" volume you are making.)*

N% stands for *New %* *(This is the "new" percent of the NV after the dilution.)*

Let's take a look at several examples to better explain what all this stuff means. You will know you are doing a dilution when you are taking a higher percent and adding a diluent like water to "dilute" it down to a lower percent or "weaker" solution. It is very important to pay attention to the wording of this kind of question so you can spot dilution problems when they appear. Otherwise, you might try to work these problems incorrectly with ratio and proportion.

Example: How many milliliters of a 20% *stock* solution of drug T would you need to prepare 500 milliliters of a 3% solution of drug T?

Solution: When reading a problem like this, you should first note that you are taking a concentrated solution (20%) and compounding a weaker solution (3%). By definition, you know this is a *dilution* and you had better **not** use ratio and proportion to solve it. You should also estimate your answer. In this example, I know that if I am making 500 ml of a weaker solution I will be using some quantity of the 20% concentrate less than 500 ml to prepare it. Now let me show you what a gazillion of my pharmacy students try to do.

Please note this is the incorrect manner to work this problem!

3%/500 ml = 20%/?

3,333 ml = ?

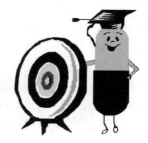

NOT EVEN CLOSE TO THE CORRECT ANSWER !!!!

Now let's work it CORRECTLY.

$$(OV)\ (O\%) = (NV)\ (N\%)$$

We want to solve for **(OV)**, or the volume of the **stock solution**. Just as with ratio and proportion, if you know three things you can easily solve for the fourth, which in this case is **(OV)**. In this and all dilution problems, you will know three factors. In this problem, you know: **(O%)** is equal to 20%, **(NV)** is 500 ml, and **(N%)** is 3%.

Now, just plug everything into the "magical" formula and solve for the missing number:

$$(OV)\qquad (O\%)\qquad =\qquad (NV)\qquad (N\%)$$

$$(OV)\qquad (20\%)\qquad =\qquad (500\ ml)\qquad (3\%)$$

$$(OV)\ =\ (500\ ml)(3\%)/(20\%)$$

$$(OV)\ =\ 1500\ ml\%/20\%$$

$$(OV)\ =\ 75\ ml$$

The 75-ml answer means you would measure 75 ml of the 20% stock solution, and *add* enough water to it *to make* 500 ml of a 3% solution.

Now I have three questions to see if you really understand the example we just solved. *Cover the correct solutions,* and try to answer these as well as you possibly can.

Question:
1

Approximately how much water will you add to the 20% solution of drug T to make this dilution?

Answer:

Approximately 425 ml of water must be *added*. If the final volume is 500 ml and you are going to use 75 ml of the 20% stock solution, then 500 minus 75 equals 425 ml. The reason I say *approximate* is because you are going to take the 75 ml of 20% and **qs** (add enough water) to make 500 ml. The true volume may be a little more or a little less than 425, but this is close enough!

Question:
2 Which volume has more of drug T in it, 75 ml of the 20% *or* 500 ml of the 3%?

Answer: Both volumes will have *exactly* the same amount of the drug in them. Do not forget, the 500-ml solution was prepared from the 75 ml, so whatever amount of drug was in the 75 ml is also in the 500 ml. If you still do not believe me, check your answers as a percent using ratio and proportion.

For the 75 ml of 20% :   20 g **drug T**/100 **ml** = ?/75 **ml**

                                            15 g **drug T** = ?

For the 500 ml of 3% :   3 g **drug T**/100 **ml** = ?/500 **ml**

                                            15 g **drug T** = ?

Question:
3 Since the 75-ml and 500-ml solutions each contain 15 g of drug T, there would also be the same amount of drug T in a teaspoon of each solution.

TRUE or FALSE?

Solution: The answer is a really big **false**. Even though both solutions, the 75 ml and the 500 ml, contain the same amount of drug, the *concentrations* of drug T are very different. One solution contains 15 g of drug in 75 ml, and the other has 15 g in 500 ml.

The **concentrated** solution would contain: 15 g **drug T**/75 **ml** = ?/5 **ml**
                                            1 g **drug T** = ?

This means there will be 1 g of drug T in each teaspoon of *concentrate*.

The **diluted** solution would contain: 15 g **drug T**/500 **ml** = ?/5 **ml**
                                            0.15 g **drug T** = ?

This means there will be 0.15 g of drug T in each teaspoon of the *dilution*.

Now let's try a few more questions using our formula, but solving for other missing factors. Again, please try to work these before looking at the solution.

Question: What is the percent sucrose in a solution if 100 ml of 50% sucrose is diluted to a pint with water?

Solution: (OV) (O%) = (NV) (N%)

(100 ml) (50%) = (480 ml) (N%)

5000 ml%/480 ml = (N%)

10.42% = N%

Question: What is the percent sucrose in a solution if 100 ml of 50% sucrose is added to a pint of water?

Did I just ask you this same question?

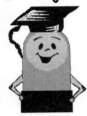

(If you said yes, then I suckered you into a common error many people make. In the first question, the final volume is 480 ml, but in this question the final volume is 580 ml because I said you added 100 ml to 480 ml. If I did not trick you here, then you are far brighter than my average student!)

The message is: READ CAREFULLY.

Solution: (OV) (O%) = (NV) (N%)

(100 ml) (50%) = (580 ml) (N%)

5000 ml%/580 ml = (N%)

8.62% = N%

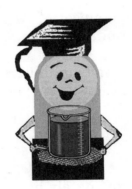

PRACTICE

11. A fluid ounce of 10% boric acid is diluted to a liter with water.

  (a) What is the percent strength of the dilution?

  (b) What is the ratio strength of the dilution?

  (c) How much boric acid is in a tablespoonful of the dilution?

  (d) How much boric acid was in a teaspoonful of the concentrated solution before the dilution was made?

12. You have 4 fluid ounces of 10% aluminum acetate solution available in your pharmacy as a stock solution.

  (a) How many milliliters of a 1:100 solution of aluminum acetate can be prepared from the volume you have on hand?

  (b) Approximately how much water would you *add* to the stock solution to prepare the dilution in Question 12a?

13. How many milliliters of a 17% benzalkonium chloride stock solution would be needed to prepare a liter of a 1:200 solution of benzalkonium chloride?

14. How many milligrams of benzalkonium chloride are in a fluid ounce of the dilution prepared in Question 13?

15. What is the percent strength of a stock solution if you took 10 ml of the stock solution and diluted it to a liter with water and had a final dilution strength of 0.5%?

16. How many grams of chemical would be in a pint bottle of the stock solution in Question 15?

17. You have a 4-ounce tube of a 5% sulfur ointment available. If you were to take 1 ounce of the sulfur ointment and *add* 4 ounces of white petrolatum (0%),

(a)   What would be the percent strength of your new diluted ointment?

(b)   What is the ratio strength of the new ointment?

18. How many milliliters of a 1:50 stock solution of an antiseptic are required to prepare a quart of a 1:2000 solution?

19. How many milliliters of water must be *added* to a pint of 95% alcohol to prepare a diluted 20% solution?

20. You have on hand 100 ml of concentrated dextrose injection 50%.

    (a)   What is the resulting percent of dextrose if you *mixed* the dextrose injection with 400 ml of water for injection?

    (b)   How much 5% dextrose could be prepared from the dextrose injection?

    (c)   How much water for injection would have to be *added* to prepare the solution in Question 20b?

    (d)   What would be the percent strength of dextrose if you *added* the concentrated dextrose to a liter bag of normal saline (0.9% NaCl)?

▼▼▼▼▼ *The answers to all problems can be found in the answer key starting on page 160.* ▼▼▼▼▼

Alligation Alternate

This section deals with a method you will not have to use very often, but it is a good procedure to know. This method is known as alligation alternate. Many of my students get confused at this point because they do not understand one very simple concept. The concept is that all of our previous dilutions were done with diluents that were 0% in strength. Some examples of these are water, white petrolatum, and, in Question 20d, the 0.9% NaCl solution.

What?

You are probably asking yourself how in the world a 0.9% NaCl solution could be 0%. The "normal saline" is 0.9% sodium chloride, but it is 0% dextrose. It is also 0% sulfur, 0% borate, 0% penicillin, 0% garlic, 0% cyanide, and 0% bedbugs.

Get the message?

The reason it is important to understand that we have been diluting with diluents that are 0% is because now we are going to dilute with diluents that are not 0%. I myself have used this process only several times because about 99% of all dilutions are simple. Now a question before we continue.

Question: If I mix 30 g of 1% hydrocortisone cream with 30 g of 2% hydrocortisone cream, I will have 60 g of a 3% hydrocortisone cream. **TRUE or FALSE?**

Solution: This is absolutely **false**. You will have 60 g of a hydrocortisone cream that has an intermediate strength somewhere between 1% and 2%. In this case, 1.5% is the strength of your new hydrocortisone mixture.

In this section, we will be using the alligation alternate method for solving dilutions made by mixing two products of known strengths to create a new product that has a percent strength somewhere between the two products being mixed. Please remember that the strength of the new product cannot be lower than the lowest percent you are mixing or higher than the highest percent.

For example, if you were to mix a 20% dextrose solution with a 5% dextrose solution, your new percent strength has to be somewhere between the strengths mixed. The new strength cannot be more than 20% and cannot be less than 5%. This may seem goofy, but it is a concept that many people, including some licensed professionals, do not grasp. To add insult to injury, I have met practitioners who sincerely believe if you put twice as much 1% ointment on your skin, you will get the same results as applying a 2% ointment. This is definitely not true!

Please remember that you should use the (OV)(O%) = (NV)(N%) method when diluting with a diluent that is 0 percent, but you should never use that method when diluting with two or more compounds that have a percent strength greater than 0. For this second kind of dilutions, use alligation alternate.

This new technique can also be used for questions with 0% diluents, but I do not recommend using it for such problems.

In the *alligation alternate* method for diluting, you will solve for the *proportional number of parts* of each component to be mixed.

All of the parts added together will equal the "whole" product you have made from the dilution. This probably makes absolutely no sense at this time, so hang in there and I will explain it further very soon.

The following steps will help you better understand the *alligation alternate* process:

Step 1.   Make three vertical columns side by side.

Step 2.   In the column to the far left, place the percent concentrations of the components to be *mixed* with the highest percent above the lowest. It will be helpful to space these two percents about 2 inches apart.

Step 3.   In the center column, place the desired percent of the compound you wish to make. Situate this percent between the percents of the two components to be *mixed,* even though they are in the left column.

Step 4.   In the column to the far right, place the numbers that reflect the *differences* in strength when you subtract the percents of the components (left column) from the desired percent (center column). There are five very important things to remember:

    ☐ You need to subtract *diagonally.*

    ☐ You must disregard positive and negative signs.

    ☐ Your answers will be in *parts* and have **no** unit value.

    ☐ The parts reflect the proportion of the components in the left column that are horizontally on line with them. They are **not** related to the component that has been subtracted.

    ☐ The total of all parts equals the amount of new product you are preparing.

Step 5.   Perform calculations using basic ratio and proportion. Remember that the *total* of **all** the parts equals the amount of the product you are trying to prepare. I am stressing this point because you must understand this concept before you start setting up your ratio and proportion equations.

Now that you are probably totally confused, let's take a look at some examples.

I promise these problems are not as hard as they sound. Follow all these steps, and you might even find them to be fun!

Example: In what proportion should a 5% ointment and a 15% ointment be mixed to prepare an 8% ointment?

Solution: Because we are mixing two ointments to compound an *intermediate*-strength product, we will need to use the alligation alternate method for diluting. Carefully follow the steps we just discussed, relating them to this example.

15% ⟵ **3 parts** (of the 15% solution)
8%
5% ⟵ **7 parts** (of the 5% solution)

Step 1. Make three vertical columns.

Step 2. Place percents of components to be mixed in left column (with 15% on top).

Step 3. Place the percent of the new compound (i.e., 8%) in the center.

Step 4. Subtract *diagonally,* place the differences in the right column, and label these numbers as *parts.* Your answer means you will mix **3 parts** of the **15%** ointment with **7 parts** of the **5%** ointment. After mixing these, you will have 10 parts of the new 8% ointment. Remember that the term parts just gives us a proportional value. We will place a unit value on the parts in our next example, so hang in there for a few more minutes.

Example: In the previous example, how much of the 15% ointment would be required to prepare 1 lb of the 8% ointment?

Solution: This may look difficult at first, but it's a piece of cake! If the *whole* amount of the 8% ointment is *10 parts* (3 parts + 7 parts), then we can say 10 parts is equal to 454 g. Now just set up a ratio and proportion with 3 parts representing the 15% ointment.

10 **parts**/454 g = 3 **parts**/?

136.2 g = ?

This means you will need to use 136.2 grams of the 15% ointment.

Question: In the previous example, how much of the 5% ointment will be needed?

Solution: Again, all you need to do is a simple ratio and proportion.

10 **parts**/454 g = 7 **parts**/?

317.8 g = ?

This means you will need 317.8 grams of the 5% ointment.

Did you notice a possible shortcut?

What is the sum of all the parts? Hopefully, it is 454 grams, because we were preparing a pound of 8% ointment. Take a minute and check our answer.

$$
\begin{array}{lll}
7 & parts\ of\ 5\% & =\ 317.8\,g \\
+\ 3 & \textbf{\textit{parts}}\ of\ 15\% & =\ \textbf{\textit{136.2 g}} \\
\hline
10 & parts & 454\,g\ \ (the\ total\ amount\ of\ 8\%\ ointment)
\end{array}
$$

So what is the possible shortcut?

Answer: If you are making 454 grams of a product and you solve for one of the two components that is going to be mixed with another component, just subtract the one component from the "whole" weight of the product to find the weight of the second component. In this example, we first determined the weight of the 15% ointment to be 136.2 grams. If the total weight is going to be 454 grams, then all you need to do is subtract **454 g – 136.2 g = *317.8 g*** to get the weight of the 5% ointment required to compound this product.

Example: From the same example, how much 8% ointment could you prepare if you have 60 grams of 5% ointment and plenty of the 15% ointment?

Solution: Do a simple ratio and proportion using the 5% as the base since it is in limited supply. Again, the 8% (i.e., final product) is represented by "10 parts."

7 **parts**/60 g = 10 **parts**/?

85.7 g = ?

Now you try to solve a couple of questions before we tackle the big problems!

Question: Continuing with the same example, what if I were to ask you how much of the 15% ointment would be mixed with 50 grams of 5% ointment to prepare the 8% ointment **(which I am getting very tired of!)?**

Solution: All you need to do is say, "If 7 parts equals 50 grams, then 3 parts equals **?**"

7 **parts**/50 g = 3 **parts**/?

21.43 g = ?

This means you would mix 21.43 grams of the 15% ointment with 50 grams of the 5% to get a final weight of 71.43 grams of 8% ointment. **Pretty cool, huh!**

Question: Now that you are the alligation master, let's see if you remember how to perform an *alligation medial* to check the previous question. Hopefully, you will come up with an average of 8% for the ointment!

Solution: Using *alligation medial:*

50.00 g	×	5%	= 250.00 g%
21.43 g	×	15%	= 321.45 g%
71.43 g			**571.45 g%**

571.45 g%/71.43 g = **8%**

Specific Gravity

Most pharmacy practitioners rarely use specific gravity in compounding, but it is a topic you need to be aware of just in case a question or need arises. Specific gravity can be defined as the ratio (written as a decimal) of the weight of a substance to the weight of an equal volume of another substance determined to be the standard. We use water as our standard for liquids and solids. Water has a specific gravity of "1," which means that 1 ml of water weighs 1 gram (at standard temperature and pressure).

Why do we need specific gravity? Because there will be times when you need to know the weight of a liquid or the volume of a solid, especially when you are compounding. The specific gravity for most substances can be found in pharmacy references.

Rules for Solving Specific Gravity Problems

When solving for the weight of a liquid, multiply the volume in milliliters of the liquid times the specific gravity and change your answer from milliliters to grams.

Example: What is the weight of a pint of chloroform (sp gr = 1.48)?

Solution: 480 ml × 1.48 = ***710.4 grams***

When solving for the *volume* of a substance, *divide* the weight of the substance in grams by the specific gravity, and change your answer from grams to milliliters.

Example: What is the volume of 200 g of a chemical (sp gr = 0.87)?

Solution: 200 g/0.87 = ***230 milliliters***

Question: How many kilograms would 2 liters of sorbitol (sp gr = 1.29) weigh?

Solution: 2000 ml × 1.29 = 2580 g = ***2.58 kg***

Question: What volume in liters would 8 lb of glycerin (sp gr = 1.25) occupy?

Solution: 454 g × 8 = 3632 g   3632 g/1.25 = 2906 ml = ***2.906 liters***

PRACTICE

21. In what proportion would a 6% ointment be mixed with a 50% ointment to prepare an ointment that has the ratio strength of 1:25?

22. A 95% alcohol is mixed with 45% alcohol to make a 55% alcohol dilution.

   (a)   In what proportions should the alcohol be mixed?

   (b)   How much of the 95% alcohol would be required to prepare a liter of the 55% alcohol?

   (c)   Using your answer to Question 22b, how much 45% alcohol would be required to prepare the mixture?

   (d)   How much of the 55% mixture can be prepared by mixing 45% and 95% alcohol solutions if you only have a pint of 95% alcohol and 3 gallons of the 45% alcohol?

23. You are asked to prepare a 1:20 coal tar ointment by combining a 1:50 coal tar ointment with pure coal tar (assume 100%).

(a)   In what proportions should the ointment and pure coal tar be mixed?

(b)   How many grams of the 1:50 coal tar ointment would be required to prepare 1 lb of the 1:20 coal tar ointment?

(c)   From your answer to Question 23b, how much pure coal tar will be needed?

(d)   How many kilograms of the 1:20 ointment could be prepared from $\frac{1}{4}$ pound of pure coal tar (assuming an unlimited supply of the coal tar ointment)?

24. For some crazy reason, you receive an order for 12% potassium chloride solution and all you have are 10% and 20% potassium chloride solutions.

(a)   In what proportion would the 10% and 20% potassium chloride solutions be mixed to prepare the 12% solution?

(b)   How many milliliters of 10% potassium chloride solution would be required to prepare a pint of the 12% solution?

(c)   How many grams of potassium chloride would be in a pint bottle of the 12% potassium chloride solution?

(d)   How many milligrams of potassium chloride would be in a tablespoonful dose of the 12% potassium chloride solution?

(e)   If you only have 20% potassium chloride solution available, how many milliliters of a diluent (0% potassium chloride) would be required to prepare a liter of the 12% potassium chloride solution?

25. You have both 1:5 and 1:100 lidocaine HCl solutions available.

(a)   Theoretically, can a 2% lidocaine HCl solution be made by mixing the two solutions?

(b)   What would be the percent strength of a solution if you mixed equal volumes of the two lidocaine solutions?

(c)   What would be the percent strength of a solution made by mixing the contents of a 30-ml vial of the 1:100 lidocaine with a 20-ml vial of a 1:5 lidocaine solution?

(d)   Lidocaine HCl is available for IV infusion in a liter solution. The label on this solution says that it contains *0.4% lidocaine HCl in 5% dextrose.* How many milligrams of lidocaine HCl will be in 1 ml of this solution?

(e)   How many grams of dextrose would a patient receive in 24 hours if she received 30 ml/hr of the solution in Question 25d?

▼▼▼▼▼ *The answers to all problems can be found in the answer key starting on page 160.* ▼▼▼▼▼

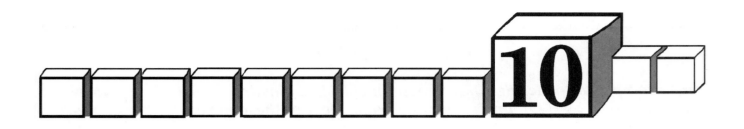

ELECTROLYTE SOLUTIONS

I have discovered over the years that the subject of electrolyte solutions and, more specifically, milliequivalents, has the tendency to strike fear in the hearts of most students and practitioners. Fortunately, as a pharmacy technician, you will rarely have to deal with solving problems related to milliequivalents unless you are in some very specialized practice setting. Also, most electrolyte solutions have both the "milligram" strength and "milliequivalent" strength on their labels.

Since you may have a limited background in chemistry, I will strive to follow my promise to K.I.S.S. (Please turn back to the Preface if you have forgotten what this means.) And, if you happen to have a Ph.D. in chemistry, please forgive me for oversimplifying a complicated subject!

OBJECTIVES

Upon mastery of Chapter 10 you will be able to:

Understand the meaning and significance of electrolyte solutions.
Recognize the valence of selected ions.
Understand atomic weight and calculate molecular weight.
Define a milliequivalent.
Solve problems related to electrolyte solutions.

All living cells are made up of atoms and molecules. The human body not only is composed of atoms, but also runs on them. I guess you could technically say we are "atomic" powered machines. All of us have countless atoms such as sodium, potassium, calcium, magnesium, chloride, oxygen, and hydrogen that are constantly moving in and out of our cells and body. These atoms frequently combine with other atoms due to bonding by electrical charges, forming molecules.

Getting Molecular

Some examples of molecules are potassium chloride, dihydrogen oxide (i.e., water, also referred to as H_2O), and sodium chloride. Most of these molecules break apart when put into solutions, forming particles known as ions. An example is when sodium chloride (NaCl) is put into water; it dissociates (i.e., breaks apart) into sodium (Na) and chloride (Cl) ions. The sodium has a positive (+) charge and the chloride has a negative (–) charge. Because of this, we say that ions carry an electrical charge and are **electrolytes**.

Some molecules, such as dextrose and urea, do not dissociate in body water. We refer to these as **nonelectrolytes**. Both electrolytes and nonelectrolytes are critical to the operation and maintenance of the human body. When they are out of balance due to disease, dehydration, and other causes, the human body can fail to function appropriately, resulting in serious illness and even death.

Throughout this textbook, we have discussed many examples and worked numerous problems related to electrolytes and nonelectrolytes. When I mentioned potassium chloride solutions, normal saline solutions, and IVs with dextrose in water, we were actually addressing electrolyte and nonelectrolyte products.

Every day in pharmacy practice you will fill prescriptions for replacement therapy. These will range from tablets to liquids to intravenous solutions. Let's take a few minutes to review a little more about electrolytes, atoms, and molecules.

For your sanity and mine, I am going to limit the scope of our discussion to just a few atoms and molecules that you will encounter frequently in everyday pharmacy practice. There are many others, but we cannot cover them all, which I am sure breaks your heart!

Each atom has an atomic weight (weights can be found in various textbooks). When atoms combine to form molecules, their molecular weight can be calculated by simply adding the atomic weights of the atoms in the molecule.

Here are some properties of common elements:

Element	Formula	Atomic Weight	Valence
Aluminum	Al	27	+3
Calcium	Ca	40	+2
Chloride	Cl	35.5	−1
Ferrous	Fe	56	+2
Hydrogen	H	1	+1
Magnesium	Mg	24	+2
Potassium	K	39	+1
Sodium	Na	23	+1

There are numerous other ions that are combinations of atoms bonded tightly together. Common examples of this kind of ion are:

Ions and Formulas		Weight	Valence
Ammonium	(NH_4)	18	+1
Acetate	$(C_2H_3O_2)$	59	−1
Bicarbonate	(HCO_3)	61	−1
Carbonate	(CO_3)	60	−2
Citrate	$(C_6H_5O_7)$	189	−3
Gluconate	$(C_6H_{11}O_7)$	195	−1
Lactate	$(C_3H_5O_3)$	89	−1
Phosphate	(H_2PO_4)	97	−1
	(HPO_4)	96	−2
Sulfate	(SO_4)	96	−2

So what is all this valence stuff?

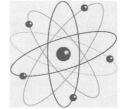

This is oversimplifying a complicated topic, but think of ions as magnets. The positive and negative poles attract and the poles that are of the same charge push apart. With this in mind, let's think about several molecules you are familiar with and see how the different charges interact.

Examples: *Sodium chloride (NaCl)* – Notice from your table that sodium has a (+1) valence (or *charge*) and chloride has a (−1) valence, so the 2 atoms combine (or *attract*), creating a molecule known as sodium chloride.

Potassium chloride (KCl) – Same concept as NaCl, with potassium (+1).

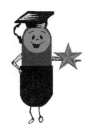

Calcium chloride (?) – Looking at the table, you will notice that calcium has a valence of (+2), so how many chlorides (−1) do you think the calcium ion would attract? If you said 2, then you get a gold star! The molecule calcium chloride has 1 calcium atom and 2 chloride atoms and is written $CaCl_2$.

Now you try several of these to see if you are catching on!

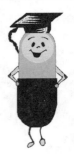

Question: How many sodium ions would be attracted to one sulfate ion?

Solution: Because the sulfate ion (SO_4) has a (–2) valence, it will attract 2 sodium ions and is properly written as Na_2SO_4.

Question: How many calcium ions do you think would be in calcium carbonate?

Solution: The calcium ion has a (+2) valence and the carbonate has a (–2) valence, so only one ion of calcium will bind with one ion of carbonate, i.e., $CaCO_3$.

Question: How many gluconate ions would be in a molecule of calcium gluconate?

Solution: The calcium ion has a valence of (+2) and the gluconate ion has a valence of (–1), so the calcium will attract 2 gluconate ions. The molecular structure will look like this: $Ca(C_6H_{11}O_7)_2$ or $C_{12}H_{22}CaO_{14}$.

Question: What would be the structure of aluminum chloride?

Solution: Because the aluminum ion has a valence of (+3), it will attract 3 chloride ions (–1). The molecular structure will be $AlCl_3$.

Question: What is the structure of magnesium sulfate?

Solution: Because magnesium has a valence of (+2) and sulfate is (–2), then 1 ion each will attract. The molecular structure is $MgSO_4$.

Note

In some products, you will have the *hydrated* form of chemicals, which means there are water molecules, i.e., H_2O attached (examples would be $CaCl_2 . 2H_2O$ and $MgSO_4 . 7H_2O$). I think this is going beyond the information you need for everyday practice, but it is important to know if there are *waters of hydration* attached. If there are, you **must** count them as part of the molecular weight of the molecule when solving for milliequivalents.

Milliequivalents (mEq)

The concentration of electrolytes in a solution is frequently expressed in units known as milliequivalents and abbreviated mEq. It is a unit of measurement of the amount of chemical activity of an electrolyte. Again, I am oversimplifying this concept to make it easier for you to understand.

Please refer to a chemistry textbook if you have a burning desire for more detail and scientific explanations and if I have insulted your intelligence. This chapter should adequately prepare you for most mEq problems without your having to search far and wide for more stimulating explanations!

What in the world is a milliequivalent and how can it be measured?

Electrolytes and nonelectrolytes normally are ordered by the physician in either *milligrams* or *milliequivalents*. I think the best way to explain milliequivalents is by relating them directly to milligrams, which you are already familiar with.

Step 1.   Calculate the atomic or molecular weight of an element and consider the weight to be milligrams. *Examples*: sodium = 23 mg and chloride = 35.5 mg, so the weight of sodium chloride would be 23 mg + 35.5 mg = **58.5 mg**.

This is not the actual weight of a molecule of sodium chloride. It is actually the weight of a millimole of sodium chloride, but that is another complicated story for another time!

Step 2.   Now take the atomic or molecular weight (expressed in milligrams) and *divide* that number by the **highest** valence of its two ions (disregard the positive or negative signs).

Let's look at several examples since this has probably totally confused you!

Example: How many milligrams are in a milliequivalent of sodium?

Step 1.   The atomic weight (AW) of sodium is 23 (call this 23 mg).

Step 2.   Since sodium has a valence of +1, divide 23 mg by 1. There are 23 mg of sodium in a mEq of sodium (i.e., 23 mg/1 = 23).

Example: How many milligrams are in a milliequivalent of calcium?

Step 1.   The atomic weight of calcium is 40 (call this 40 mg).

Step 2.   Since calcium has a valence of +2, divide 40 mg by 2. There are 20 mg of calcium in a mEq of calcium (i.e., 40 mg/2 = 20).

Example: How many milligrams are in a milliequivalent of potassium chloride?

Step 1.   The molecular weight of KCl is $39 + 35.5 =$ **74.5 mg.**

Step 2.   Since the two valences are +1 and −1, disregard the sign and just divide 74.5 mg by 1. This means there are 74.5 mg potassium chloride in a milliequivalent of KCl (i.e., 74.5 mg/1 = 74.5).

Example: How many milligrams are in a milliequivalent of calcium chloride?

Step 1.   The molecular weight of $CaCl_2$ is 111. This is a little different from the previous examples because there are 2 chloride ions and 1 calcium ion ($35.5 + 35.5 + 40 =$ **111 mg**).

Step 2.   The chloride ions have a valence of −1, and the calcium is +2. Divide 111 mg by 2 (i.e., the largest valence regardless of sign). There are 55.5 mg in a mEq of $CaCl_2$ (i.e., 111 mg/2 = 55.5).

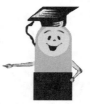

Note   As mentioned earlier, if the calcium chloride is in the *hydrated* form, it will have the structure $CaCl_2 .2H_2O$, and the molecular weight will be 147. A milliequivalent of the *hydrated* calcium chloride will be 147 mg/2 = 73.5 mg.

Example: How many milligrams are in a milliequivalent of potassium citrate?

Step 1.   The molecular weight of $C_6H_5K_3O_7$ is 306.
Citrate ($C_6H_5O_7$) = 189 and 3 potassiums = $3 \times 39 =$ **117**
for a total molecular weight of $117 + 189 =$ **306 mg.**

Step 2.   The 3 potassium ions each have a valence of +1 and the citrate ion is −3. Divide 306 mg by 3 (i.e., the largest valence regardless of sign). There are 102 mg in a milliequivalent of potassium citrate (i.e., 306 mg/3 = 102 mg).

Remember this concept: Whenever you have a milliequivalent of any compound, you can make a statement of unity which is,"1 milliequivalent of the molecule yields upon dissociation 1 mEq of each of the ions that made up the original molecule."

Example: In the last example, we determined there are 102 milligrams of potassium citrate per milliequivalent of potassium citrate. We can say that **1 mEq** of **potassium citrate** (i.e., 102 mg) yields upon dissociation 1 mEq of **potassium** ion and 1 mEq of **citrate** ion.

Now I realize this might not make a lot of sense, but trust me on this one because it is getting late and I am hungry!

How can you use this statement of unity in practice?

Example: How much potassium citrate would provide 5 mEq of potassium?

Solution: Based on our *statement of unity* just discussed, **1** mEq of potassium is contained in **1** mEq of potassium citrate. By using basic logic, we know that **5** mEq of potassium would be contained in **5** mEq of potassium citrate. Now, by using ratio and proportion, solve for the answer in milligrams. Remember from the last example that there were 102 mg of potassium citrate/milliequivalent.

102 mg K-citrate/1 mEq K-citrate = ?/5 mEq K-citrate

510 mg potassium citrate = ?

This means you would give the patient 510 mg of potassium citrate which is the same as giving 5 mEq of potassium citrate or 5 mEq of potassium, which is just what the doctor ordered!

Now it is your turn to try a tough one!

Question: What would be the percent strength of a sodium bicarbonate injection if the label on a vial reads 0.9 mEq sodium bicarbonate per milliliter?

Solution:

Step 1.   The molecular weight of sodium bicarbonate equals 84.

Step 2.   84 mg/1 = 84 mg sodium bicarbonate per mEq sodium bicarbonate.

To solve for a percent, just convert (mEq/ml) to (mg/ml) to (grams/100 ml).

1 mEq sod. bicarb./84 mg sod. bicarb. = 0.9 mEq sod. bicarb./?

75.6 mg sodium bicarbonate = ?

This means there are 75.6 mg of sodium bicarbonate per ml **or** 7,560 mg/100 ml: 7,560 mg/100 ml → 7.56 g/100 ml → *7.56% solution of sodium bicarbonate.*

PRACTICE

1. A patient has a prescription for one pint of 10% potassium chloride liquid.

    (a)　　　　How many grams of potassium chloride (KCl) are in the bottle?

    (b)　　　　How many milliequivalents of potassium chloride are in the bottle?

    (c)　　　　How many mEq of *potassium* are in the bottle?

    (d)　　　　How many mEq of potassium chloride are in a tablespoonful dose?

    (e)　　　　How many milliliters of this solution would a patient receive daily if her physician orders 10 mEq of *potassium* q.i.d.?

2. A professional football player takes 1-gram sodium chloride (NaCl) tablets during the hot summer days in football camp.

    (a)　　　　How many milliequivalents of sodium chloride are in each tablet?

    (b)　　　　How many mEq of *sodium* does he receive from these tablets in a week if he takes 1 tablet t.i.d.?

    (c)　　　　If his trainer wants him to receive 100 mEq of *sodium* each day, how many tablets should he take?

3. How many grams of sodium chloride would be required to prepare a liter of a solution containing 154 mEq of sodium chloride?

4. What is the percent strength of the solution in Question 3?

5. A physician likes to write orders for patients to receive 1 mEq of *sodium* per kilogram of body weight.

  (a)   How many milligrams of sodium chloride would a 72-kg patient receive?

  (b)   How many grams of sodium chloride would a 110-pound patient receive?

  (c)   How much normal saline (0.9% NaCl)) would provide the sodium chloride for the patient in Question 5b?

  (d)   How many milliliters of concentrated 14.6% sodium chloride injection would provide the sodium for the patient in Question 5b?

6. If a patient receives 100 ml of 5% dextrose and normal saline (D_5NS) every hour, how many milliequivalents of *sodium* will she receive in 24 hours?

7. You receive an order to prepare a solution containing 30 mEq of calcium/L.

  (a)   How many milligrams of calcium chloride ($CaCl_2$) would be required to prepare this solution? (Let's use a MW = 111.)

  (b)   What would be the percent concentration of calcium chloride in this solution?

8. You are asked to prepare a solution of sodium bicarbonate to contain 90 mEq of *sodium* per 100 ml.

    (a)   How many milligrams of sodium bicarbonate ($NaHCO_3$) would be needed to prepare a liter of this solution?

    (b)   What is the percent concentration of sodium bicarbonate in this solution?

9. The directions on a vial of ammonium chloride say to add a 20-ml vial of ammonium chloride containing 100 mEq of ammonium chloride to 500 ml of normal saline.

    (a)   What is the percent strength of ammonium chloride (NH_4Cl) in the vial?

    (b)   What is the percent of ammonium chloride when added to the 500 ml of normal saline?

10. Sodium acetate injection is available in 50-ml vials containing 4 mEq/ml.

    (a)   How many milliliters would provide a 1-gram dose?

                Sodium acetate = $NaC_2H_3O_2$ MW = 82   Valence = 1

    (b)   How many milliequivalents of *sodium* are in 5 ml of injection?

    (c)   What is the percent strength of sodium acetate in this solution?

▼▼▼▼▼ *The answers to all problems can be found in the answer key starting on page 160.* ▼▼▼▼▼

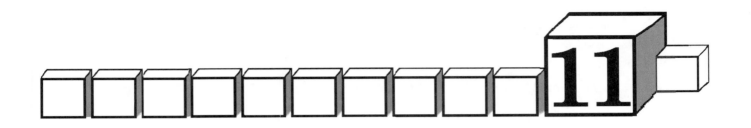

TEMPERATURE CONVERSIONS

*I*n 1709, Gabriel D. Fahrenheit, a German physicist, invented an alcohol thermometer. *Seven years later he improved his thermometer by using mercury instead of alcohol. The scale he used on the improved thermometer indicated that (at sea level) water started to freeze at 32° and water started to boil at 212°. This was the beginning of the Fahrenheit scale for measuring temperature. It has been used in many parts of the world for centuries and is the primary measure of temperature used in the United States.*

Several decades after Fahrenheit's scale was established, a Swedish astronomer named Anders Celsius suggested a more convenient thermometer based on water starting to freeze at 0° and starting to boil at 100°. We are now faced with the reality that some people use the Fahrenheit (°F) scale and others use the Celsius or centigrade (°C) scale when measuring temperature. (Does this sound a lot like our chapter on "conversions"?) For your sanity and mine, I am going to make this a really short chapter (sweet and simple)! All you really need to know is how to convert back and forth.

OBJECTIVES

Upon mastery of Chapter 11 you will be able to:

Explain the differences between the Fahrenheit and centigrade scales.
Convert degrees centigrade to degrees Fahrenheit.
Convert degrees Fahrenheit to degrees centigrade.

There are two or three formulas commonly used for converting between the Fahrenheit and centigrade (Celsius) systems. You may be familiar with some that use fractions such as $\frac{9}{5}$, $\frac{5}{9}$, and 0.55. For the sake of simplicity, I want you to learn only what I consider the easiest and least confusing formulas and forget about those "common" fractions.

The How-to Stuff

To convert from centigrade to Fahrenheit: °F = (1.8 × °C) + 32

To convert from Fahrenheit to centigrade: °C = (°F − 32) ÷ 1.8

Example: Convert 100°C (the boiling point of water) to degrees Fahrenheit.

You should already know this answer based on our previous discussion, but let's try it and see if our formula really works.

Solution:
°F = (1.8 × °C) + 32
°F = (1.8 × 100°) + 32
°F = (180°) + 32
°F = ***212°***

Example: Do you remember at what centigrade temperature water freezes? If you do not remember, I'll give you a hint that it is 32°F. Now plug this information into your other formula, and see if the formula works.

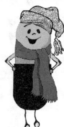

Solution:
°C = (°F − 32) ÷ 1.8
°C = (32° − 32) ÷ 1.8
°C = (0°) ÷ 1.8
°C = ***0°***

Now you try to solve a couple of these questions.

Question: A baby's rectal temperature is measured with a thermometer to be 102°F. Express this temperature in degrees centigrade.

Solution:
°C = (°F − 32) ÷ 1.8
°C = (102° − 32) ÷ 1.8
°C = (70°) ÷ 1.8
°C = ***38.9°***

Question: Would you put on a sweater if the temperature sign at your neighborhood bank said it was 49°C?

Solution:
°F = (1.8 × °C) + 32
°F = (1.8 × 49°) + 32
°F = (88.2°) + 32
°F = ***120.2°***   **I hope you do not need a sweater!**

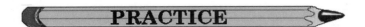 **PRACTICE**

1. Convert the following Fahrenheit temperatures to degrees centigrade.

   (a)   41°F

   (b)   86°F

   (c)   167°F

   (d)   14°F

   (e)   − 40°F

2. Convert the following centigrade temperatures to degrees Fahrenheit.

   (a)   15°C

   (b)   75°C

   (c)   0°C

   (d)   − 5°C

   (e)   − 75°C

▼▼▼▼▼ *The answers to all problems can be found in the answer key starting on page 160.* ▼▼▼▼▼

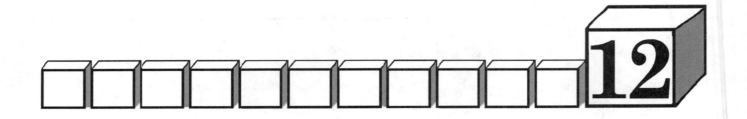

BUSINESS MATH

*W*e are coming down the "home stretch," but even though you are the master of practically everything you need to know in pharmacy math, you still need to learn about the marketing or business aspects of pharmacy practice. I think every pharmacy you work in is likely to have its own approach to pricing and discounting, and there are many variations in business math. In this last chapter, we will look at basic terms and procedures so you will be able to function in the "business" world of pharmacy.

OBJECTIVES

Upon mastery of Chapter 12 you will be able to:

Define commonly used business terms in pharmacy practice.
Calculate markup prices and percents.
Determine sale or discount prices.
Compute net profit and gross profit.
Estimate inventory turnover rates.

Common Business Terms

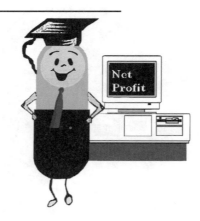

Here are some basic business terms you ought to know:

AWP – *Average Wholesale Price* is the published "theoretical" price a pharmacy pays for a medication, theoretical because pharmacies normally pay less than AWP due to discounts, contracts with wholesalers, special deals, group purchasing, etc.

Markup – The difference between merchandise cost and the selling price of an item.

Gross margin – Also referred to as *gross profit,* this is the difference between the selling price and the acquisition (purchase) price; usually refers to the total inventory.

Overhead – The expenses associated with doing business, e.g., rent, utilities, and salaries.

Net profit – The true profit after all associated expenses are subtracted. This would be the gross profit minus overhead expenses.

Markdown – Also referred to as *discounts* and *sales*. This is a reduction of a set price.

Inventory – An itemized list of the merchandise and cost in a particular establishment.

Turnover rate – How often the total inventory is sold over a specific time period.

Markup

Markup is a term that is often used interchangeably with gross margin and gross profit. If you purchase a television set from a local retailer for $189 and the retailer paid $150 to the manufacturer for the television, then the retailer's *markup* is $39.

Markup = selling price − cost

$39 = $189 − $150

Question: What would be the markup on an antibiotic a pharmacy purchased from a wholesaler for $25 and sold to a patient for $32?

Solution: **Markup = selling price − cost**

$7 = $32 − $25

Percent Markup

Percent markup (percent of gross margin) is the percent determined by dividing the markup by the **selling price** or, in some cases, dividing by the **cost** of the merchandise. It is very important for you to clarify what the *percent markup* is based on. Let's use the last example to determine percent markup by both *selling price* and *cost*.

Percent markup = selling price − cost/*selling price*
*(based on **selling price**)*

= ($32 − $25)/$32

= $7/$32 = 0.219 = **21.9%** percent markup (based on ***selling price***)

Percent markup = selling price – cost/cost
(based on cost)

$$= (\$32 - \$25)/\$25$$

$$= \$7/\$25 = 0.28 = \textbf{28\%}\ \text{percent markup (based on \textit{cost})}$$

Question: What is the percent markup based on *selling price* of a laxative that cost the pharmacy $3.50 and is sold to a patient for $5.50?

Solution: % markup = $5.50 – $3.50/$5.50

% markup = $2.00/$5.50 = 0.36 = **36%** markup (based on selling price)

Question: In the previous question, what is the percent markup based on *cost*?

Solution: % markup = $5.50 – $3.50/$3.50

% markup = $2.00/$3.50 = **57%** markup
(based on cost)

Question: A pharmacy purchases a sunscreen from a wholesaler for $5. Store policy is to mark up all nonprescription products 45% based on *cost*. What will be the selling price after the markup?

Solution: You are going to have to think about this a little bit before calculating. Some people like to solve for 45% of $5, which is $2.25, and then add the numbers together to get a selling price of **$7.25**. I like to simply multiply the cost ($5) times a factor of 1.45 (i.e., 145%) to get $7.25.

Question: Using the last example, what would be the price if store policy was to mark up all nonprescription products by 45% based on the *selling price*?

Solution: *Please note that this problem is worked differently from the previous one.* If the markup is 45% of the selling price, then the *cost* would be 55% (100% – 45% = 55%). Again, you can solve by ratio and proportion.

55%/100% = $5/?

$9.09 = ?

Note

You can see that there is a big difference in the final cost to a consumer depending on whether the 45% fee is based on **cost** or on **selling price**.

Percent Discounts

Percent discounts (markdowns or sales) occur when there is a reduction in the original selling price of an item. (Discounts also can be given by the wholesaler when a pharmacy pays its bills within a certain timeframe.) These discounts are almost always based on *selling price* and can be solved in a similar manner as our last example which was also based on *selling price*.

Example: Let's pretend you go to the mall for an after holiday sale and see an $80 outfit on sale for 33% off the ticketed price. How much would the outfit cost after the discount?

Solution: If 100% of the price is $80, then you will only have to pay 67%. In other words, 100% original price – 33% discount = 67%.

67%/100% = ?/$80

$53.60 = ?

Question: The pharmacy you work at is selling humidifiers for 25% off. What would a humidifier originally priced at $35 cost after the markdown is taken off?

Solution: Consider the original price, $35, to be 100%. The price after the sale is 75% of the original price (100% – 25% = 75%).

100%/75% = $35/?

$26.25 = ?

Gross Profit

Although *gross profit (gross margin)* is similar to markup, it usually is used to refer more to the big picture of store sales. Markup is generally associated with individual products. *Gross profit* is the difference between total sales minus the cost of items sold.

Example: If a store has sales totaling $2,000,000 and the cost of the items sold is $1,500,000, then the *gross profit* is $500,000 (i.e., sales – cost = gross profit).

Net Profit

Net profit is what some people affectionately call the bottom line. This is the true profit store owners are concerned with. The difference in *net* profit and *gross* profit is that *net profit* subtracts from total sales **both** the cost of goods sold **and** overhead.

Example: Using the previous example for gross profit, what is the net profit if overhead expenses (i.e., security, rent, electricity, insurance, technician's *high* salaries) total about $350,000?

Solution: Net profit = sales − (cost of goods + overhead)

Net profit = $2,000,000 − ($1,500,000 + $350,000)

Net profit = $2,000,000 − $1,850,000

Net profit = $150,000

As mentioned earlier, gross and net profits can be used to analyze annual sales, monthly sales, and even a single prescription. Also, many store owners study various departments within a store (cosmetics, durable medical equipment, nonprescription drugs, etc.) to establish which areas produce the best profits and which are performing poorly.

Inventory Turnover Rate

Most pharmacies take an *inventory* (a count of all store items and their cost) at least once a year. Inventory *turnover* is the frequency with which items sell over a specific period. The *inventory turnover rate* can be determined by taking the cost of **all** goods purchased during a period of time and dividing this number by the average cost of the pharmacy inventory.

Example: During the past 12 months, a pharmacy spent $1,800,000 on inventory purchases. Average inventory value during the past year was determined to be $300,000. What was the *inventory turnover rate*?

Solution: Inventory turnover rate = total purchases/average inventory

Inventory turnover rate = $1,800,000/$300,000 = **6 times**

The more turnovers of inventory a store has the better. High turnover rates indicate that you are not investing too much money in inventory that is just sitting on the shelf looking pretty, depreciating, and possibly going out of date.

PRACTICE

1. A patient buys a pair of crutches for $78 that the pharmacy purchased from a durable medical equipment supplier for $45.

   (a)   What is the markup on the crutches?

   (b)   What is the percent markup of the crutches based on selling price?

   (c)   What is the percent markup of the crutches based on cost?

   (d)   What would be the price on a pair of crutches if the supplier's price remained the same, but the store owner decided to charge a 72% markup based on cost?

   (e)   Considering the scenario in Question 1d, what would be the new price if the 72% markup is based on the selling price?

2. The markup on 60 antidepressant tablets is $12 and a patient pays $78 for the entire prescription.

   (a)   What was the acquisition cost of the tablets for the pharmacy?

   (b)   What was the average cost to the patient for each tablet?

(c)   What was the markup on each tablet?

(d)   If the patient takes 1 tablet bid, what will the cost be to the patient for a week of antidepressant therapy?

(e)   What was the percent markup of the prescription based on cost?

(f)   What was the percent markup based on selling price?

3. A pharmacy accountant reported this information after an annual inventory:

Total annual overhead expenses = $850,000
Total inventory purchases = $2,670,000
Total sales = $4,300,000
Average inventory = $520,000

(a)   What was the gross profit for this establishment?

(b)   What was the net profit for this store?

(c)   If the owner decided to give her pharmacy technician 5% of the net profit, how much would this be and would you accept it?

(d)   What was the inventory turnover rate?

(e)   Approximately how many sales took place if the average sale was $62?

4. The prescription department had the following monthly sales information:

> Net profit = $5,328
> Total sales receipts = $81,435
> Total drug costs = $69,887

(a)   What was the gross profit for the month?

(b)   What was the overhead for the month?

5. A 100-tablet bottle of a new cardiovascular drug cost the pharmacy $331.

(a)   How much would 30 tablets cost a patient with a 20% markup
         based on acquisition cost?

(b)   How much would 60 tablets cost a patient with a 10% markup
         based on selling price?

(c)   The wholesaler gives the pharmacy an 8% discount if all debts
         are paid in full in 30 days. How much would the bottle of 100 tablets
         cost if the pharmacy qualifies for the discount?

▼▼▼▼▼ *The answers to all problems can be found in the answer key starting on page 160.* ▼▼▼▼▼

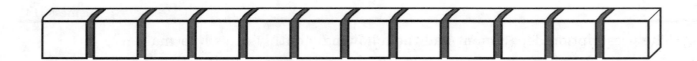

POSTTEST:
MEGA MATH MARATHON

It has been a pleasure helping you overcome the barriers associated with learning pharmaceutical calculations. If you have mastered the material in this textbook you will be able to answer the majority of questions you will encounter in pharmacy practice.

This last section is designed to give you a chance to solve real world problems and evaluate how knowledgeable you have become about pharmacy math. Please work the following problems slowly and carefully. Do not work these questions until you have mastered <u>all</u> the objectives in this textbook. You have been prepared for each of these 101 questions (events), but in some cases you will have to search a little to find the information you need (molecular weights, labeling information, for example).
Read every question carefully. I will constantly attempt to see if I can trick you into making a careless error. When you finish this posttest, add up all your correct "event" answers and score yourself as follows:

GOLD MEDAL (90–101): **You are awesome!**

SILVER MEDAL (80–89): **You should be very proud of yourself!**

BRONZE MEDAL (70–79): **You are doing well, but you could do better!**

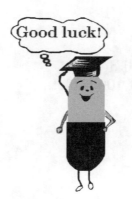

If you score below 70, you need to practice, practice, practice. Then return to this chapter and try again. Hopefully you will be in contention for a medal next time.

Just remember, *you* are a *winner* for studying and for trying to improve your skills.

I WISH YOU THE BEST OF LUCK IN YOUR PHARMACY CAREER.

NOW, LET THE MARATHON BEGIN!

For events 1–3:

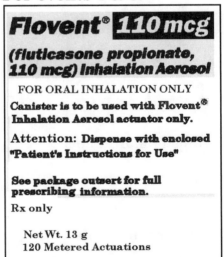

Canine Diarrhea Capsules

R/ *(For 100 capsules)*

Neomycin sulfate	1.44 g
Sulfaguanidine	14.8 g
Sulfadiazine	920 mg
Sulfamerazine	920 mg
Sulfathiazole	920 mg
Kaolin	30 g
Pectin	1 g

Courtesy of *International Journal of Pharmaceutical Compounding*

1. How many milligrams of neomycin sulfate are contained in 1 capsule?

2. What is the percent strength of neomycin sulfate in this formula?

3. How many milligrams of kaolin would be required to prepare 30 capsules?

For events 4 & 5:

Flovent® 110 mcg
(fluticasone propionate, 110 mcg) Inhalation Aerosol

FOR ORAL INHALATION ONLY

Canister is to be used with Flovent® Inhalation Aerosol actuator only.

Attention: Dispense with enclosed "Patient's Instructions for Use"

See package outsert for full prescribing information.

Rx only

Net Wt. 13 g
120 Metered Actuations

4. How many milligrams of fluticasone propionate are in a canister?

5. What is the percent strength of fluticasone propionate in this canister?

For events 6 & 7:

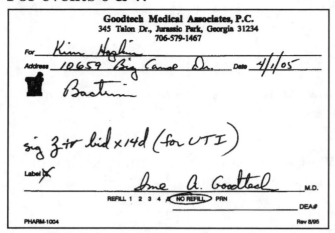

6. How many milliliters of Bactrim® suspension would you dispense?

7. Bactrim suspension contains 200 mg of sulfamethoxazole and 40 mg of trimethoprim per 5 ml. How many total grams of the drugs will Kim receive daily?

For events 8 & 9:

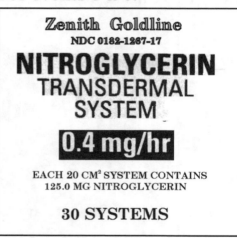

8. How many micrograms of nitroglycerin will a patient receive in 12 hours?

9. How many grams of nitroglycerin are in all of the systems in this box?

For events 10–12:

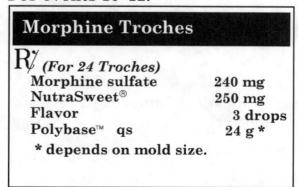

Courtesy of *International Journal of Pharmaceutical Compounding*

10. How many milligrams of morphine are in each troche?

11. What is the mg% of morphine sulfate in this formulation?

12. How many grams of NutraSweet® are required to prepare 100 troches?

For events 13–15:

USUAL DOSAGE: Apply to the affected area as a thin film from two to four times daily depending on the severity of the condition. Store at controlled room temperature 15°- 30°C (59°-86°F). Avoid excessive heat above °C (104°F) See package insert for full prescribing information. E. FOUGERA & CO. a division of Altana Inc. MELVILLE, NEW YORK 11747b NDC 0168-0139-30 **fougera** ® **FLUOCINONIDE** **CREAM USP, 0.05%**	To Open: To puncture the seal, reverse the cap and place the puncture-top onto the tube. Push down firmly until seal is open. To close, screw the cap back onto the tube. CAUTION: Federal law prohibits dispensing without prescription. WARNING: Keep out of reach of children. FOR EXTERNAL USE ONLY. NOT FOR OPHTHALMIC USE. KEEP CONTAINER TIGHTLY CLOSED. NET WT 30 grams

13. How many milligrams of fluocinonide are in three tubes of this cream?

14. What would be the percent strength of fluocinonide in a cream prepared by mixing a tube of this cream with 60 grams of a cream containing no fluocinonide?

15. In °C, above what temperature is considered "excessive heat"?

For events 16–19:

PLEASE USE BALL POINT PEN – PRESS FIRMLY

GOODTECH MEMORIAL HOSPITAL

WRITE OR IMPRINT PATIENT INFORMATION BELOW

GENERIC EQUIVALENT MAY BE DISPENSED UNLESS CHECKED ☐

DATE	HOUR	PHYSICIANS ORDERS	DO NOT USE THIS SHEET UNLESS RED NUMBERS SHOWS ①
		Vitals q/hr	
4/1/05	1735	Seizure precautions	
		Begin MgSO4 infusion at 4gm/hr and cont.	
		for 24 hours	
		Serum 7, Mg++ in AM	
		Minnie Goodtech MD	

16. You are directed to mix 20 g of $MgSO_4$ in 500 ml D_5W. The $MgSO_4$ is supplied in 2-ml vials of 50% solution. How many vials are needed to prepare the 500-ml order? (NOTE: Volume adjusted to 500 ml.)

17. At what rate would the nurse set the infusion pump to provide the ordered dose of magnesium sulfate?

18. What is the drip rate in gtt/min if the infusion set delivers 20 gtt/ml?

19. To be prepared to supply the entire order, how many bags are needed?

For events 20 & 21:

ROCEPHIN® (ceftriaxone sodium) FOR INJECTION

500 mg   Single Use Vials

Directions for Use:
For I.M. Administration: Reconstitute with 1.0 mL 1% Lidocaine Hydrochloride Injection (USP) or Sterile Water for Injection (USP). Each 1 mL of solution contains approximately 350 mg equivalent of ceftriaxone.
For I.V. Administration: Reconstitute with 4.8 mL of an I.V. diluent specified in the accompanying package insert. Each 1 mL of solution contains approximately 100 mg equivalent of ceftriaxone.
Withdraw entire contents and dilute to the desired concentration with the appropriate I.V. diluent.
Storage Prior to Reconstitution: Store powder at room temperature 77° F (25° C) or below.
Protect From Light.
Storage After Reconstitution: See package insert.
USUAL DOSAGE: For dosage recommendations and other important prescribing information, read accompanying insert.
ROCHE LABORATORIES INC., Nutley, New Jersey 07110

---

20. What is the dry powder volume based on the directions for I.V. administration?

21. According to the <u>I.M.</u> directions for administration, how many milliliters of the reconstituted solution would provide a 200-mg dose of Rocephin®?

For events 22–24:

Acyclovir Stick with Sunscreen	
R *(For five 5-g tubes)*	
Acyclovir 200-mg capsules	5 capsules
Para-aminobenzoic acid	150 mg
Silica gel, micronized	120 mg
Polyethylene glycol 3350	6.5 g
Polyethylene glycol 300	15 mL

Courtesy of *International Journal of Pharmaceutical Compounding*

22. How many grams of acyclovir would be required to prepare 10 tubes?

23. How many grams of para-aminobenzoic acid are in each tube?

24. How many milligrams of silica gel are in 1 gram of this formulation?

For events 25 & 26:

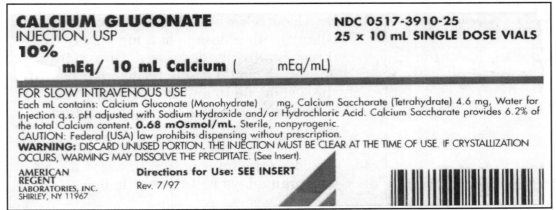

CALCIUM GLUCONATE
INJECTION, USP
10%

NDC 0517-3910-25
25 x 10 mL SINGLE DOSE VIALS

mEq/ 10 mL Calcium (mEq/mL)

FOR SLOW INTRAVENOUS USE
Each mL contains: Calcium Gluconate (Monohydrate)   mg, Calcium Saccharate (Tetrahydrate) 4.6 mg, Water for Injection q.s. pH adjusted with Sodium Hydroxide and/or Hydrochloric Acid. Calcium Saccharate provides 6.2% of the total Calcium content. **0.68 mOsmol/mL.** Sterile, nonpyrogenic.
CAUTION: Federal (USA) law prohibits dispensing without prescription.
WARNING: DISCARD UNUSED PORTION. THE INJECTION MUST BE CLEAR AT THE TIME OF USE. IF CRYSTALLIZATION OCCURS, WARMING MAY DISSOLVE THE PRECIPITATE. (See Insert).

AMERICAN
REGENT
LABORATORIES, INC.
SHIRLEY, NY 11967

Directions for Use: SEE INSERT
Rev. 7/97

25. How many milliequivalents of calcium would be contained in a vial if calcium gluconate has a molecular weight of 430 and a valence of 2?

26. How many milligrams of calcium gluconate are in all the vials in this package of single-dose vials?

For events 27 & 28:

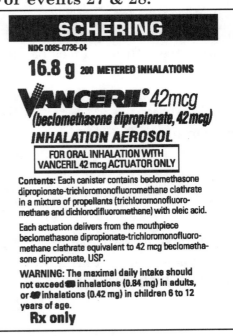

SCHERING

NDC 0085-0736-04

16.8 g 200 METERED INHALATIONS

VANCERIL® 42mcg
(beclomethasone dipropionate, 42 mcg)
INHALATION AEROSOL

FOR ORAL INHALATION WITH
VANCERIL 42 mcg ACTUATOR ONLY

Contents: Each canister contains beclomethasone dipropionate-trichloromonofluoromethane clathrate in a mixture of propellants (trichloromonofluoromethane and dichlorodifluoromethane) with oleic acid.

Each actuation delivers from the mouthpiece beclomethasone dipropionate-trichloromonofluoromethane clathrate equivalent to 42 mcg beclomethasone dipropionate, USP.

WARNING: The maximal daily intake should not exceed ⬤ inhalations (0.84 mg) in adults, or ⬤ inhalations (0.42 mg) in children 6 to 12 years of age.

Rx only

27. How many inhalations are considered maximal for an adult?

28. What is the mg% strength of beclomethasone in Vanceril® aerosol?

For events 29–31:

Progesterone 50-mg/mL Topical Gel	
Progesterone, micronized	5 g
Hydroxyethylcellulose	3 g
Alcohol, 95%	35 mL
Purified water qs	100 mL

Courtesy of *International Journal of Pharmaceutical Compounding*

29. What is the percent alcohol in the final product?

30. What is the percent progesterone in 1 tablespoonful of this gel?

31. How many grams of hydroxyethylcellulose would be required to prepare 4 fluid ounces of this gel?

For events 32 & 33:

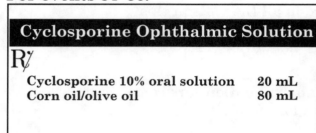

Goodtech Medical Associates, P.C.
345 Talon Dr., Jurassic Park, Georgia 31234
706-579-1467

For _Angie Hopkins_

Address _95601 Big Canoe Dr._   Date _4/1/05_

℞   Dilantin – 125

℥ viii

Sig. tid

Label ✗

Ane A. Goodtech   M.D.

REFILL 1 2 3 4 5 NO REFILL (PRN)

DEA#

32. Dr. Goodtech wants Angie to receive the Dilantin® in a dosage of 5 mg/kg/day in three equally divided doses. How many milliliters would Angie receive per dose if she weighs 66 lb and the Dilantin-125 suspension contains 125 mg phenytoin per tsp?

33. Based on the information in event 32, how many days will the bottle last?

For events 34–36:

Cyclosporine Ophthalmic Solution	
℞	
Cyclosporine 10% oral solution	20 mL
Corn oil/olive oil	80 mL

Courtesy of *International Journal of Pharmaceutical Compounding*

34. What is the percent strength of cyclosporine in this product?

35. How many milliliters of cyclosporine would be required to prepare 2 fluid ounces of this formulation?

36. How many milligrams of cyclosporine are in 1 ml of this formulation?

For events 37 & 38:

Case:
A patient named Ace Goodtech purchases a triamcinolone acetonide aerosol inhaler for $68.85. The physician has directed Ace to use two inhalations 3 times a day. The label on the product indicates it is a 20 g inhaler and contains 240 metered actuations. Ace is leaving town today on a two-week vacation.

37. How many inhalations will Ace use while he is on vacation, assuming he is compliant with his physician's directions?

38. What will be the cost for the amount of medication inhaled while Ace is on vacation?

For events 39 & 40:

Prior to Reconstitution: Store at a Controlled Room Temperature 20° to 25°C (°to °F.) Protect from light.
After Reconstitution: *Kefzol* is stable for 24 hours at room temperature **Usual Adult Dose:** 250 mg to 1 gram every 6 to 8 hours. To prepare I.V. solution - See accompanying prescribing information for directions. Each ADD-Vantage® Vial contains: 1 gram of cefazolin. The sodium content is 48 mg per gram of cefazolin. For use only with ADD-Vantage® Flexible Diluent Container. ADD-Vantage® (Vials and diluent containers, Abbott Laboratories) ℞only

39. What is the temperature range in degrees °F for storage of Kefzol®?

40. How many milliequivalents of sodium will a patient receive in 3 days from Kefzol if he takes 1 gram of Kefzol q8h? (AW sodium = 23, valence = 1)

For events 41–44:

ADULT PARENTERAL NUTRITION ORDERS

ADDRESSOGRAPH

** ALL TPN ORDERS MUST BE IN THE PHARMACY BY 2:00 P.M. DAILY. VOLUMES ORDERED WILL BE INFUSED OVER 24 HOURS.

1) CONSULT NUTRITIONAL SUPPORT SERVICE

2) Check formulation desired:	*STANDARD CENTRAL	MODIFIED CENTRAL	**STANDARD PERIPHERAL	MODIFIED PERIPHERAL	
AMINO ACIDS	70 gms		70 gms		*Standard Central formulation contains: 70gms protein, 420 gm dextrose, 1708 kcals excluding lipids (NOTE:Day 1 formulation will contain 210gms dextrose & 994 kcals) rate= 62ml/hr Na 99mEq, Cl 98mEq, K 70mEq,Ca 14mEq, Mg 24mEq, PO4 18mM, Acetate 135mEq
DEXTROSE	420 gms		140 gms		
VOLUME (mls)	1500 mls		2000 mls		
NaCl			40 mEq		
(Na) Phosphate	18 mM		9 mM		
Na Acetate	75 mEq		70 mEq		
KCl	70 mEq		40 mEq		
(K) Phosphate					**Standard Peripheral formulation contains: 70gms protein, 140gms dextrose, 686 kcals excluding lipids. rate=84ml/hr Na 122mEq, Cl 108mEq K 40mEq, Mg 10mEq, PO4 9mM, Acetate 131mEq
K Acetate					
Ca Gluconate	14 mEq		7 mEq		
Mg Sulfate	24 mEq		10 mEq		
MVI-12	10 mls		10 mls		
M.T.E.-4	3 mls		3 mls		
Vitamin K	1 mg		1 mg		
Other					

41. How many milliliters of an 8.5% amino acid solution would be required to provide the amino acids for a standard central TPN order?

42. If the dextrose in the standard central TPN is provided by 600 ml of a dextrose solution, what is the percent of the 600 ml of dextrose?

43. How many milligrams of calcium gluconate (MW = 430, valence = 2) are required to prepare a standard peripheral TPN?

44. How many milliliters of a 1-g/10-ml calcium gluconate solution would provide the calcium gluconate needed for event 43?

For events 45–47:

Testosterone Propionate Gel		
R/ *(For 100 g)*	2%	3%
Testosterone propionate	2 g	3 g
Mineral oil, light	10 g	10 g
Polysorbate 80	1 g	1 g
Methylcellulose 2% gel	87 g	86 g

Courtesy of *International Journal of Pharmaceutical Compounding*

45. How many grams of testosterone would be required to prepare 1 lb of the 3% gel?

46. What is the percent strength of methylcellulose in the 2% formulation?

47. How many milliliters of light mineral oil (sp gr 0.84) would provide the weight ordered in either of the formulas?

For events 48 & 49:

20 AMPULS

METHERGINE®
(methylergonovine maleate)
injection, USP

1 ml **(0.2** mg**)** SIZE

Each 1 ml contains:
methylergonovine maleate, USP .... 0.2 mg (1/320 gr)
   Inactive Ingredients
tartaric acid, NF .... 0.25 mg
sodium chloride, USP .... 3 mg
water for injection, USP, qs to .... 1 ml

Usual dose: One ml intravenously or intramuscularly after delivery of anterior shoulder, after delivery of the placenta, or during the puerperium. See package insert for further dosage information.

CAUTION: Federal law prohibits dispensing without prescription.

SandoPak® (unit dose pack)   6505-00-116-1374

48. How many µg of tartaric acid would be in 3 doses of Methergine®?

49. How many milliequivalents of sodium chloride would be contained in all of the ampuls in this package? (MW NaCl = 58.5, valence = 1)

For events 50 & 51:

INDICATIONS: Helps treat and prevent diaper rash. Protects chafed skin due to diaper rash and helps protect from wetness. Also helps to prevent and temporarily protect chafed, chapped, cracked, or windburned skin and lips.
DIRECTIONS: Change wet and soiled diapers promptly, cleanse the diaper area, and allow to dry. Apply **DIAPER RASH Ointment** liberally as often as necessary, with each diaper change, especially at bedtime or anytime when exposure to wet diapers may be prolonged.
ACTIVE INGREDIENT: Zinc Oxide 40%.
INACTIVE INGREDIENTS: Cod Liver Oil (High in Vitamins A & D), Petrolatum, BHA, Fragrance, Lanolin, Methylparaben, Talcum, and Purified Water.

DIAPER RASH OINTMENT NDC 45802-179-44

A RECOMMENDED DIAPER RASH FORMULA
AND SKIN PROTECTANT
PROTECTS SKIN, RELIEVES CHAFING
NET WT. 4 OZ. (113 g)

50. How many kilograms of zinc oxide would the manufacturer need to prepare 1,000 lb of this diaper rash ointment?

51. The pricing code at this pharmacy puts the cost of the product on the second line of the pricing label and leaves out the decimal places. The cost of this diaper rash ointment is 104 or $1.04. What is the percent markup based on cost if the retail price to customers is the price on the bottom line of the attached sticker?

For events 52–54:

Nystatin Popsicles®

R︎ *(For 10 popsicles®)*

Nystatin powder	2,500,000 units
Sorbitol 70% solution	20 mL
Syrup, NF	50 mL
Flavoring (banana,	5 mL
or other flavor to taste)	
Purified water qs	300 mL

Courtesy of *International Journal of Pharmaceutical Compounding*

52. What is the percent sorbitol in the final solution?

53. What is the percent volume-volume of the banana flavoring?

54. How many units of nystatin are in 2½ Popsicles?

For events 55–57:

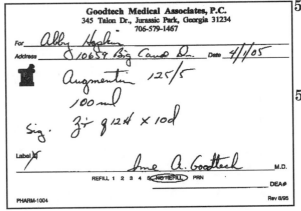

Goodtech Medical Associates, P.C.
345 Talon Dr., Jurassic Park, Georgia 31234
706-579-1467

For _Abby Hopkin_
Address _10659 Big Camp D._ Date _4/1/05_

Augmentin 125/5
100 ml
Sig. 3ⁱ q12h x 10d

Label ☑

Ime A. Goodtech M.D.

REFILL 1 2 3 4 5 NO REFILL PRN

DEA#

PHARM-1004   Rev 8/95

55. The label on the bottle of Augmentin® says to reconstitute with 90 ml of water. What is the dry powder volume displacement?

56. If you accidentally reconstituted this prescription with 100 ml of water, how many milliliters of the incorrectly reconstituted Augmentin would provide the appropriate dose? (NOTE: In real life you would probably pour this mistake down the sink and start over.)

57. Approximately how many pounds would Abby weigh if the package insert for Augmentin recommends a dose of 30 mg/kg/day?

For events 58 & 59:

50 ampuls 2 mL each   NDC 0173-0260-35

LANOXIN® (digoxin)
Injection

500 mcg (0.5 mg) in 2 mL
(250 mcg [0.25 mg] per mL)

Store at 25°C (77°F); excursions permitted to 15 to 30°C (59 to 86°F) [see USP Controlled Room Temperature] and protect from light.

58. A physician orders a loading dose of digoxin to be 250 mcg I.V. q6h for 1 day. How many single-dose ampuls will be required?

59. A physician orders an I.V. digitalizing dose of 30 mcg/kg for a 14-lb baby. How many milliliters of the Lanoxin® injection should be given?

For events 60–62:

```
Veterinary Electrolyte Injection
Rx
  Sodium acetate trihydrate        4.333 g
  Potassium chloride               467 mg
  Calcium chloride dihydrate       200 mg
  Magnesium chloride               133 mg
  Benzyl alcohol                   0.1 mL
  5% Dextrose in water             50 mL
  Sterile water for injection   qs 100 mL
```

Courtesy of *International Journal of Pharmaceutical Compounding*

60. How many milliequivalents of potassium are in this formulation? (AW potassium = 39, MW potassium chloride = 74.5, valence = 1)

61. What is the percent dextrose in the final solution?

62. How many milliequivalents of magnesium chloride are in this formulation? (MW $MgCl_2$ = 95, valence = 2)

For events 63–65:

GOODTECH MEMORIAL HOSPITAL			WRITE OR IMPRINT PATIENT INFORMATION BELOW
GENERIC EQUIVALENT MAY BE DISPENSED UNLESS CHECKED ☐			
DATE	HOUR	PHYSICIANS ORDERS	DO NOT USE THIS SHEET UNLESS RED NUMBERS SHOWS.
4/1/05	1530	1) Obtain stat PTT, PT, CBC (if not already done) 2) Give bolus dose of heparin 5000 units IV 3) Heparin 25,000 units in 500 ml ½ NS at 800 units/hr via pump. Begin infusion at same time as heparin bolus dose. 4) Bleeding precautions 5) PTT 6 hours p̄ heparin therapy begins 6) Daily CBC + PTT	
		Minnie Goodtech MD	

63. The "bolus" dose of heparin is based on 75 units/kg of body weight. How many pounds does this patient weigh?

64. How many milliliters per hour will be given via pump to provide the patient with the prescribed heparin infusion?

65. If an I.V. set delivers 15 gtt/ml, how many gtt/min would provide the appropriate heparin dose, assuming a pump is not available and the I.V. set had to be utilized?

For events 66 & 67:

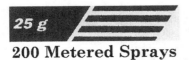

NDC 0173-0388-79

GlaxoWellcome

Beconase AQ®
(beclomethasone
dipropionate,
monohydrate)
Nasal Spray, 0.042%*

25 g

200 Metered Sprays

Spray — For Intranasal Use Only
* Calculated on the dried basis.

Caution: Federal law prohibits
dispensing without prescription.

Important: Read accompanying
directions carefully.

66. How many milligrams of beclomethasone dipropionate are in this canister?

67. How many micrograms of beclomethasone dipropionate are in two intranasal sprays?

For events 68–70:

Cocaine-Phenol-Tannic Acid Ointment	
R℞ *(For 100 g)*	
Cocaine hydrochloride	1.5 g
Phenol crystals	3 g
Tannic acid	10 g
Hydrous lanolin	40 g
White petrolatum qs	100 g

Courtesy of *International Journal of Pharmaceutical Compounding*

68. How much white petrolatum is required to prepare this product?

69. What is the ratio strength of cocaine in this formulation?

70. How many grams of phenol crystals are required to make 8 oz. of this formulation?

For events 71 & 72:

NDC 0517 - 1130 - 01
30 mL
MULTIPLE DOSE VIAL

EPINEPHRINE
INJECTION, USP

FOR SC AND IM USE
FOR IV AND IC USE
AFTER DILUTION

AMERICAN
REGENT
LABORATORIES, INC.
SHIRLEY, NY 11967

Each mL contains:
1 mg Epinephrine as the
hydrochloride, Water for
Injection, q.s. Sodium
Chloride added for
isotonicity, 0.5%
Chlorobutanol as a
preservative and not
more than 0.15% Sodium
Metabisulfite as an
antioxidant. pH may be
adjusted with Sodium
Hydroxide and/or
Hydrochloric Acid.
STORE BETWEEN
15° AND 25° C
(59° AND 77° F).
Protect from light and
freezing.
Usual Dosage: See
package insert.

71. What is the ratio strength of this epinephrine injection?

72. How many milligrams of chlorobutanol are in a vial?

For events 73 & 74:

Triple Antibiotic Ointment
(Neomycin and Polymyxin B Sulfates and Bacitracin Zinc Ointment USP)

First Aid Antibiotic

WARNINGS:
For external use only. Do not use in the eyes or apply over large areas of the body. In case of deep or puncture wounds, animal bites, or serious burns, consult a doctor. Stop use and consult a doctor if the condition persists or gets worse, or if a rash or other allergic reaction develops. Do not use this product if you are allergic to any of the ingredients. Do not use longer than one week unless directed by a doctor. Keep this and all drugs out of the reach of children. In case of accidental ingestion, seek professional assistance or contact a Poison Control Center immediately.

DIRECTIONS:
Clean the affected area. Apply a small amount of this product (an amount equal to the surface area of the tip of a finger) on the area 1 to 3 times daily. May be covered with a sterile bandage.

Each gram contains: neomycin sulfate 5 mg equivalent to 3.5 mg of neomycin base, polymyxin B sulfate equal to 5,000 polymyxin B units, and bacitracin zinc equal to 400 bacitracin units in a base of white petrolatum.

Store at room temperature.

See crimp of tube for Control No. & Exp. Date.

73. On the attached pricing label, the number 79 is the cost to the pharmacy (i.e., 79 cents) and the bottom numbers indicate the retail price to the consumers. What is the percent markup based on selling price?

74. How many units of polymyxin B are in a 1-oz tube of this ointment?

For events 75 & 76:

Usual Dosage
For dosage and other prescribing information, see accompanying product literature.

Dispense in a light-resistant container as defined in the official compendium.

Store at controlled room temperature (15°-30°C, 59°-86°F). Protect from light. Do not freeze.

Haldol®
BRAND OF
HALOPERIDOL INJECTION
(For Immediate Release)
5 mg per mL
10 x 1-mL
STERILE AMPULS

Caution: Federal law prohibits dispensing without prescription.

Each mL contains:
Haloperidol 5 mg (as the lactate) with 1.8 mg methylparaben, 0.2 mg propylparaben, and lactic acid for pH adjustment to 3.0-3.6

For Intramuscular Use

McNeil Pharmaceutical
McNeilab, Inc.
Spring House, PA 19477

© McN '93   701-94-066-4

McNEIL PHARMACEUTICAL

75. The attending physician wants his 220-lb psychotic patient to receive Haldol® 0.1 mg/kg/day in divided doses b.i.d. How many milligrams of Haldol will this patient receive per dose?

76. How many ampuls must be sent to the patient's unit to provide a week supply of the Haldol prescribed in event 75?

For events 77–79:

Piroxicam 1% Alcoholic Gel

R℞ Piroxicam   1 g
     Hydroxypropylcellulose   1.75 g
     Propylene glycol   5 mL
     Polysorbate 80   2 mL
     70% Isopropyl alcohol qs   100 mL

Courtesy of *International Journal of Pharmaceutical Compounding*

77. What is the weight of propylene glycol (sp gr 1.04) in this formula?

78. What is the percent strength of hydroxypropylcellulose in 3 quarts of this formulation?

79. How many grams of piroxicam are required to prepare a gallon of this formulation?

For events 80 & 81:

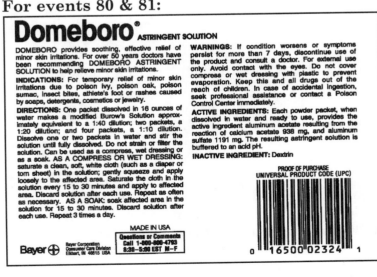

80. What is the percent of the Domeboro® dilution when 1 packet is dissolved in a pint of water?

81. How many Domeboro packets would a patient need if he is preparing 1 pint of the 1:20 dilution q.i.d. x 5 days?

For events 82 & 83:

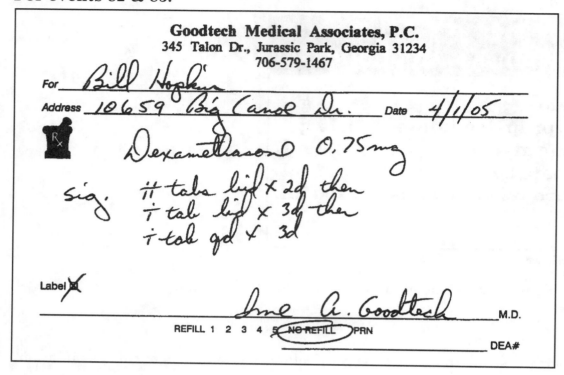

82. How many dexamethasone 0.75-mg tablets should be dispensed to properly fill this prescription?

83. How many total grams of dexamethasone will this patient receive?

For events 84 & 85:

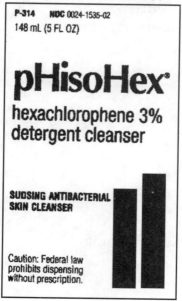

84. How many grams of hexachlorophene are in a bottle of pHisoHex®?

85. How many kilograms of hexachlorophene would be required to prepare a 20,000-liter vat of pHisoHex?

For events 86–88:

Idoxuridine Ophthalmic Solution

℞

Idoxuridine		100 mg
Thimerosal		2 mg
Sterile water for injection	qs	100 mL

Courtesy of *International Journal of Pharmaceutical Compounding*

86. What is the percent strength of idoxuridine in this formulation?

87. What is the milligram percent of thimerosal in this formulation?

88. How many micrograms of idoxuridine would be required to prepare ½ fluid ounce of this formulation?

For events 89 & 90:

NDC 0456-0672-99

7g 100 metered inhalations

AEROBID®
(flunisolide)
Inhaler System

FOR ORAL INHALATION ONLY

Contains flunisolide as the hemihydrate suspended in propellants (trichloromono-fluoromethane, dichlorodifluoromethane and dichlorotetrafluoroethane) with sorbitan trioleate as a dispersing agent.

Each activation delivers approximately 250 mcg flunisolide to the patient.

Caution: Federal law prohibits dispensing without prescription.

mfd for

FP **FOREST PHARMACEUTICALS, INC.**
SUBSIDIARY OF FOREST LABORATORIES, INC.
ST. LOUIS, MISSOURI 63045

89. The recommended dose for Aerobid® is 2 inhalations b.i.d. How many canisters should a patient purchase if he is going on a trip around the world that will last 92 days?

90. How many milligrams of flunisolide will the patient inhale during the trip around the world mentioned in event 89?

For events 91–94:

GOODTECH MEMORIAL HOSPITAL			WRITE OR IMPRINT PATIENT INFORMATION BELOW

GENERIC EQUIVALENT MAY BE DISPENSED UNLESS CHECKED ☐

DATE	HOUR	PHYSICIANS ORDERS	DO NOT USE THIS SHEET UNLESS RED NUMBERS SHOWS.
4/1/05	0800	Admit to Dr. Goodtech's service	
		Dx: pneumonia, N/V	
		CBC ō diff, SMA 7 in AM	
		Zosyn 3 gm IV q6h	
		Solu-Medrol 80mg IV q6h	
		Reglan 10-20 mg IV q6h prn N/V	
		Tylenol 325mg ī-tī po q4-6h prn pain/HA	
		Regular diet	
		Minnie Goodtech MD	

91. Solu-Medrol® is available for injection in a 125-mg/2-ml vial. How many milliliters of this injection are required for each ordered dose?

92. Reglan® injection is available in 2-ml amps containing 5 mg/ml. How many amps would supply the maximum ordered daily dose?

93. How many grams of Tylenol® would this patient receive daily if he received the maximum quantity ordered?

94. Zosyn® is reconstituted in the pharmacy to contain 3.375 g/20 ml. How many milliliters should be administered every 6 hours according to Dr. Minnie Goodtech's order to provide this patient an unusual dose?

For events 95–97:

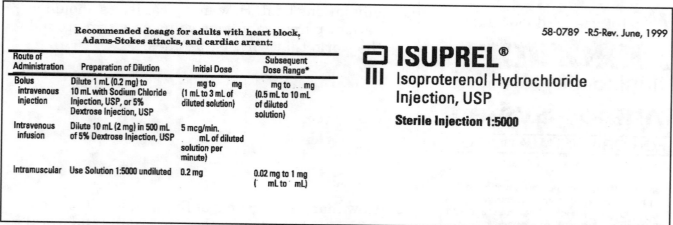

95. What is the range in milligrams of Isuprel® that a patient would receive as an initial dose from a bolus intravenous injection route of administration?

96. How many milliliters per minute of the diluted Isuprel solution would provide the initial dose from an intravenous infusion route of administration?

97. How many milliliters of undiluted Isuprel would provide the initial dose by the intramuscular route of administration?

For events 98 & 99:

Analgesic Medication Stick

R℞ *(For 100 g)*

Methyl salicylate	35 g
Menthol	15 g
Sodium stearate	13 g
Purified water	12 g
Propylene glycol	25 g

Courtesy of *International Journal of Pharmaceutical Compounding*

98. What is the ratio strength of propylene glycol in this formulation?

99. How many grams of sodium stearate are needed to make 2.75 kg of this formulation?

For events 100 & 101(our bonus question):

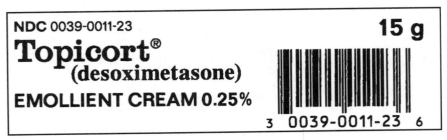

6505-00-926-2095

fougera

HYDROCORTISONE CREAM, U.S.P. 1%

CONTAINS: 10 mg of Hydrocortisone per gram in a base containing Glyceryl Monostearate, Polyoxyl 40 Stearate, Glycerin, Paraffin, Stearyl Alcohol, Isopropyl Palmitate, Sorbitan Monostearate, Benzyl Alcohol, Potassium Sorbate, Lactic Acid, and Purified Water.

NET WT. 1 OZ. (28.35g)

NDC 0039-0011-23   **15 g**

Topicort®
(desoximetasone)

EMOLLIENT CREAM 0.25%

3 0039-0011-23 6

100. How many grams of 2.5% hydrocortisone cream should be mixed with this tube of hydrocortisone to prepare a 1.25% hydrocortisone cream?

BONUS *(THIS IS REAL TRICKY!)*

101. What would be the percent strength of desoximetasone in a product prepared by mixing the tubes of hydrocortisone and Topicort®?

ANSWER KEY

CHAPTER 1

1a	200 (rule 1)
1b	No value (rule 3)
1c	3000 (rule 1)
1d	No value (rule 2)
1e	40 (rule 4)
1f	No value (rule 6)
1g	55 (rule 5)
1h	No value (rule 8)
1i	12 (rule 5)
1j	No value (rule 7)
1k	22
1l	51
1m	110
1n	150
1o	66
1p	1004
1q	515
1r	29
1s	445
1t	No answer, just seeing if you are awake.
1u	XVIII
1v	XXXIV
1w	XLVII
1x	LXII
1y	CDLXXX
1z	MCMXCIX

2a $7 \times 1/12 = 7/1 \times 1/12 = 7/12$

2b $3/5 \times 1/5 = 3/25$

2c $1\,1/6 \times 2\,½ = 7/6 \times 5/2 = 35/12 = 2\,11/12$

2d $1/500 \times 5 = 1/500 \times 5/1 = 5/500 = 1/100$

2e $8¾ \times 3/120 = 35/4 \times 3/120 = 105/480 = 21/96 = 7/32$

3a $3/5 \div 4/5 = 3/5 \times 5/4 = 15/20 = ¾$

3b $19¼ \div 3 = 77/4 \div 3/1 = 77/4 \times 1/3 = 77/12 = 6\,5/12$

3c $1/50 \div 1/200 = 1/50 \times 200/1 = 200/50 = 4$

3d $11 \div 3¾ = 11/1 \div 15/4 = 11/1 \times 4/15 = 44/15 = 2\,14/15$

3e $1/8 \div 8 = 1/8 \div 8/1 = 1/8 \times 1/8 = 1/64$

4a $3/8 + 5/16 = 6/16 + 5/16 = 11/16$

4b $9/13 + 1/3 = 27/39 + 13/39 = 40/39 = 1\,1/39$

4c $1\,5/8 + 3¾ + 5\,3/10 = 13/8 + 15/4 + 53/10 = 65/40 + 150/40 + 212/40 = 427/40 = 10\,27/40$

4d $10½ + 5 + 6\,1/3 = 21/2 + 5/1 + 19/3 = 63/6 + 30/6 + 38/6 = 131/6 = 21\,5/6$

4e $3\,2/3 + 5½ + 5/11 = 11/3 + 11/2 + 5/11 = 242/66 + 363/66 + 30/66 = 635/66 = 9\,41/66$

5a $4/5 - 3/10 = 8/10 - 3/10 = 5/10 = ½$

5b $5\,1/12 - 2/3 = 61/12 - 2/3 = 61/12 - 8/12 = 53/12 = 4\,5/12$

5c $11¾ - 9½ = 47/4 - 19/2 = 47/4 - 38/4 = 9/4 = 2¼$

5d $3/100 - 1/150 = 9/300 - 2/300 = 7/300$

5e $7\,2/5 - 2/3 = 37/5 - 2/3 = 111/15 - 10/15 = 101/15 = 6\,11/15$

6 $¾ + ½ + 2 + 1\,5/8 = ¾ + ½ + 2/1 + 13/8 = 6/8 + 4/8 + 16/8 + 13/8 = 39/8 = 4\,7/8$ pounds

7 $4\,7/8 - 1½ = 39/8 - 3/2 = 39/8 - 12/8 = 27/8 = 3\,3/8$ pounds eaten

8 $3/8 + 1½ + 3/16 + 2 = 3/8 + 3/2 + 3/16 + 2/1 = 6/16 + 24/16 + 3/16 + 32/16 = 65/16 = 4\,1/16$ lb

9 *Step 1* $3 \times 1¼ = 3/1 \times 5/4 = 15/4 = 3¾$ lb used
Step 2 $4\,1/16$ lb $- 3¾$ lb used $= 65/16 - 1\,5/4 = 65/16 - 60/16 = 5/16$ lb

10 24 teaspoons $\div ¾ = 24/1 \div ¾ = 24/1 \times 4/3 = 96/3 = 32$ doses

11 5 tablets $\times 1/150$ gr $= 5 \times 1/150 = 5/1 \times 1/150 = 5/150 = 1/30$

12 $3/16$ ounce $\div 30$ capsules $= 3/16 \div 30/1 = 3/16 \times 1/30 = 3/480 = 1/160$ oz

13a $15 + 1.5 + 0.15 + 150 = 166.65$

13b $3.25 + 13.091 + 0.18 = 16.521$

13c $0.38 + 0.097 + 0.0062 = 0.4832$

13d $22.0008 + 8.022 = 30.0228$

14a $32 - 1.0009 = 30.9991$

14b $2.52 - 0.333 = 2.187$

14c $491.08 - 321.008 = 170.072$

14d $0.0678 - 0.00678 = 0.06102$

15a $23.8 \div 0.294 = 80.952$

15b $0.91 \div 8.27 = 0.11$

15c $341.44 \div 0.37 = 922.81$

15d $68.2 \div 2000 = 0.0341$

16a $0.003 \times 0.09 = 0.00027$

16b $54.5 \times 25.12 = 1,369.04$

16c $100.25 \times 100.35 = 10,060.087$

16d $1336 \times 10,000 = 13,360,000$

17a XXIV $\times 3.25 = 24 \times 3.25 = 78$

17b $26.23 \times 6\,7/12 = 26.23 \times 6.583 = 172.68$

17c LXVI $+ 41.9 + 333\,½ = 66 + 41.9 + 333.5 = 441.4$

17d (cxiiiss) (8 3/8) $= 113.5 \times 8.375 = 950.56$

17e LXVII $-$ XLII $= 67 - 42 = 25 =$ XXV

17f $17.1 \div 4\,3/8 = 17.1 \div 4.375 = 3.91$

17g $3¾ \div 3.089 = 3.75 \div 3.089 = 1.214$

17h $5.029 \times 19\,7/8 = 5.029 \times 19.875 = 99.95$

NOTE: It is easiest to convert all common fractions to decimal fractions.

18 $96 \div 4\,4/5 = 96 \div 4.8 = 20$ salads

19 XXXII $\div 8.5 = 32 \div 8.5 = 3.76$ ounces

20 MDCXXXV $\div$ CIX $= 1635 \div 109 = 15$ technicians

21 *Step 1* (Determine how much has been dispensed.)
30 capsules $\times 1.25 = 37.50$ grams
15 capsules $\times 2.75 = 41.25$ grams
10 capsules $\times 1.5 = \underline{15.00}$ grams
93.75 grams dispensed
Step 2 100 grams $-$ 93.75 grams $= 6.25$ grams remaining

22 6.25 grams remaining $\div 1¾ = 6.25 \div 1.75 = 3.57$, but only three capsules can be completely filled.

23 $32.5 + 15\,3/8 + 75.5 + 118\,1/8 = 32.5 + 15.375 + 75.5 + 118.125 = 241.5 =$ CCXLISS

24 $¾ \div 0.00055 = 0.75 \div 0.00055 = 1363.63$

25 $\$350 \times 0.001 = \$0.35$

CHAPTER 2

1a	25 kilograms = 25,000 grams
1b	55 grams = 55,000 milligrams
1c	72 milligrams = 72,000 micrograms
1d	105 liters = 105,000 milliliters
1e	48 meters = 4,800 centimeters
1f	1,257 millimeters = 1.257 meters
1g	387 centimeters = 3,870 millimeters

1h   43 millimeters = 4.3 centimeters
1i   982 milligrams = 0.982 gram
1j   3,389 milligrams = 0.003389 kilogram
1k   0.0765 milligram = 76.5 micrograms
1l   0.00376 gram = 3,760 micrograms
1m   5,786 milliliters = 5.786 liters
1n   0.0698 liter = 69.8 milliliters
1o   0.00997 kilogram = 9,970 milligrams
1p   8,023,766 grams = 8,023.766 kilograms
1q   7,569 micrograms = 0.007569 gram
1r   355.56 milliliters = 0.35556 liter
1s   0.0298 meter = 29.8 millimeters
1t   0.002289 milliliter = 2.289 liters
1u   0.200897 kilogram = 200,897,000 micrograms

2   635 g + 0.58 kg + 428,970 mg = 635 g + 580 g + 428.97 g = 1643.97 grams

3   1.27 kg ÷ 429 grapes = 1270 grams ÷ 429 grapes = 2.96 grams each

4   454 g ÷ 22,700 mg/pot = 454 g ÷ 22.7 g/pot = 20 pots of coffee

5   1.89 L ÷ 210 ml/glass = 1890 ml ÷ 210 ml = 9 glasses

6   2.6 km × 2 = 5.2 km = 5,200 meters

7   8 lb × 454 grams/lb = 3,632 g = 3.632 kg

8   99 bandages × 7.62 cm = 754.38 cm = 7.5438 meters

9   378 g + 0.86 kg + 198,000 mg + 38,000,000 mcg = 378 g + 860 g + 198 g + 38 g = 1474 g

10   1.5 kg − 1474 g = 1500 g − 1474 g = 26,000 mg needed

11   3.84 L ÷ 120 ml/bottle = 3840 ml ÷ 120 ml = 32 bottles

12   3 kg ÷ 90 g/shaker = 3000 g ÷ 90 = 33.33 shakers or 33 "full" shakers

13   2500 capsules × 750 mcg = 1,875,000 mcg = 1,875 mg = 1.875 grams

14   0.0009 kg ÷ 30 mg/capsule = 900 mg ÷ 30 mg = 30 capsules

15   40 mg tobramycin in 1 ml = 4 mg/0.1 ml = 4,000 micrograms

16   178 cm = 1,780 mm

17a   5 qt = 5 qt × 32 ounces/quart = 160 fluid ounces
17b   3 gallons = 3 gal. × 8 pints/gallon = 24 pints
17c   498 pints = 498 pt ÷ 8 pints/gal. = 62.25 gallons
17d   322 fl.ounces = 322 fl. ounces ÷ 32 fl. ounces per quart = 10.06 quarts
17e   960 minims = 960 minims ÷ 480 minims per fluid ounce = 2 fluid ounces
17f   480 fl. drams = 480 fl. drams ÷ 8 fl. drams per fl. ounce = 60 fluid ounces
17g   ¼ gallon = ¼ gallon × 8 pints/gallon = 2 pints
17h   76 ounces = 76 ounces × 480 gr/ounce = 36,480 grains
17i   64 drams = 64 drams ÷ 8 drams/ounce = 8 ounces

NOTE: It is important to *estimate* when working all problems. *Estimation* is essential in understanding whether to multiply or divide by conversion factors. Try to *estimate* more if you had difficulty with the previous questions.

18   2 gallons ÷ 4 fl ounces per bottle = 256 fl ounces ÷ 4 fl ounces = 64 bottles

19   *Step 1*   180 gr × 7 days = 1260 grains/week
      Step 2   1260 grains ÷ 480 grains/ounce = 2.625 grains

20   1¾ ounces ÷ 1¾ gr/capsule = 840 gr ÷ 1.75 gr/capsule = 480 capsules

21a   168 lb = 168 lb × 16 oz per lb = 2,688 ounces
21b   137 oz = 137 oz ÷ 16 oz per lb = 8.56 lb
21c   36 oz = 36 oz × 437.5 gr per oz = 15,750 gr
21d   768 gr = 768 gr ÷ 7000 gr per lb = 0.1097 lb
21e   1276 gr = 1276 gr ÷ 437.5 gr per oz = 2.92 oz

22   1 1/8 lb + 15 oz + 3276 gr = 18 oz + 15 oz + 7.49 oz = 40.49 oz

NOTE: Your answers may be a little different than mine based on *conversion factors* being used. All of the following can be worked several different ways.

23a   4.5 tsp = 4.5 tsp × 5 ml per tsp = 22.5 ml
23b   325 lb = 325 lb ÷ 2.2 lb per kg = 147.7 kg
23c   3,000 gr = 3,000 gr ÷ 15.4 gr per gram = 194.81 grains
23d   289 kg = 289 kg × 2.2 lb per kg = 635.8 pounds
23e   75 ml = 75 ml ÷ 5 ml per tsp = 15 tsp
23f   67 g = 67 g × 15.4 gr per g = 1031.8
23g   6.5 lb = 6.5 lb × 16 oz per lb = 104 ounces
23h   118 mg = 118 mg ÷ 65 mg per grain = 1.82 gr
23i   727 oz = 727 oz ÷ 16 oz per lb = 45.44 lb
23j   1700 ml = 1700 ml ÷ 480 ml per pint = 3.54 pints
23k   43 gr = 43 gr × 65 mg per gr = 2795 mg
23l   35 tbsp = 35 tbsp × 3 tsp per tbsp = 105 tsp
23m   4.8 pints = 4.8 pints × 480 ml per pint = 2304 ml
23n   3 fl ounces = 3 fl ounces × 6 tsp per fl ounce = 18 tsp
23o   64 fl ounces = 64 fl ounces ÷ 16 fl ounces per pint = 4 pints
23p   111 kg = 111 kg × 2.2 lb per kg = 244.2 lb
23q   485 lb = 485 lb ÷ 2.2 lb per kg = 220.45 kg
23r   4 quarts = 4 quarts × 960 ml per quart = 3840 ml = 3.84 liters
23s   15,000 ml = 15,000 ml ÷ 3840 ml per gallon = 3.91 gallons
23t   5¾ lb = 5¾ lb × 454 g per lb = 2610.5 grams
23u   2150 ml = 2150 ml ÷ 15 ml per tbsp = 143.3 tbsp
23v   3½ oz = 3.5 oz × 28.4 g per oz = 99.4 grams

24a   18 gr + 2600 mg + 1.3 g + ¼ oz = 18 gr + 40 gr + 20 gr + 109.4 gr = 187.4 grains
24b   187.4 gr = 187.4 gr × 65 mg per gr = 12,181 mg or (12.181 g for Question 24c)
24c   ½ oz = ½ oz × 28.4 g per oz = 14.2 g in stock − 12.181 g dispensed = 2.019 g

25a   1/8 gal + ½ qt + ½ pt + 5 fl oz + 8 tbsp + 15 tsp = 480 ml + 480 ml + 240 ml + 150 ml + 120 ml + 75 ml = 1545 ml = 309 teaspoons
25b   1 gallon − 1545 ml = 3840 ml − 1545 ml = 2295 milliliters remain

CHAPTER 3

1a   4/12 = 1/3 = 0.333 = 1:3
1b   20/210 = 2/21 = 0.095 = 2:21*
*NOTE: This is the improper form for writing ratios. We will discuss the correct configuration in a future chapter.
1c   38/218 = 19/109 = 0.174 = 19:109*
1d   6/10 = 3/5 = 0.6 = 3:5*
1e   5/1000 = 1/200 = 0.005 = 1:200
1f   44/100 = 22/50 = 11/25 = 0.44 = 11:25*
1g   3/15 = 1/5 = 0.2 = 1:5
1h   30/600 = 3/60 = 1/20 = 0.05 = 1:20
1i   600/2400 = 60/240 = 6/24 = ¼ = 0.25 = 1:4

2   200 calories/2.1 oz = ?/19 oz   ? = 1809.5 calories

3   1 shampoo/5 ml = ?/750 ml   ? = 150 shampoos

4a   75 sheets/1 week = ?/42 weeks
      ? = 3150 sheets of paper per year

4b   75 sheets/1 student = ?/26 students
      ? = 1950 sheets per week

5   2.92 mg sodium/1 fl oz = ?/12 fl oz
      ? = 35.04 mg = 0.03504 gram

6   1500 rumples/$1 = 480,000 rumples/?
      ? = $320

7   12 diapers/1 day = ?/14 days
      ? = 168 diapers (whew!)

8   18 miles/8 pints (gallon) = 698 miles/?
      ? = 310.22 pints

9   1.2 mg/1 fl oz = ?/8 fl oz
      ? = 9.6 mg = 9,600 micrograms

10   1 Rx/135 seconds = ?/3600 seconds (hour)
      ? = 26.7 prescriptions per hour

11   5 mg diazepam/1 tab = ?/500,000 tabs
      ? = 2,500,000 mg = 2.5 kg

12   25 mg expect./15 ml (tbsp) = ?/960 ml (quart)
      ? = 1,600 mg expectorant per quart

13   182 lb sulfur/$2134 = 3 lb/?   ? = $35.18

14   20 mg antiflatulent/0.3 ml = ?/30 ml
      ? = 2,000 mg = 2 g antiflatulent

15   5 gr ASA/1 tablet = ?/250 tablets
      ? = 1,250 gr = 81.17 grams ASA

16   10 g ZnO/100 g oint. = 170.25 g ZnO/?
      ? = 1,702.5 grams of ointment
      (3/8 pound = 3/8 × 454 g = 170.25 g)

17   1 kg/2.2 lb = ?/186 lb   ? = 84.55 kg

18   0.25 mg alpr./1 tab = ?/100 tabs
      ? = 25 mg = 0.385 grain

19   960 mg med/480 ml (pint) = ?/10 ml (2 tsp)
      ? = 20 mg = 0.02 gram

20   **NOTE: 1/150 gr = 0.00667 gr**
      0.00667 gr/1 tablet = ?/30 tablets
      ? = 0.2 grain = 13 mg

21   1.4 ml/1 minute = ?/1440 minutes (1 day)
      ? = 2,016 ml = 2.016 liters

22   0.75 mg (750 mcg)/1 vial = 15 mg/?
      ? = 20 vials

23    $32/3840 ml (gal) = ?/1000 ml   ? = $8.33

24   2270 g sugar/3000 ml = ?/5 ml   ? = 3.78 grams sugar

25   130 mg (2 gr)/90 capsules = ?/1 capsule
      ? = 1.444 mg or 1,444 mcg

CHAPTER 4

1a   Put (instill) 3 drops in right eye every 6 hours as needed for pain.

1b   One tablet under the tongue (sublingually) as needed for shortness of breath.

1c   Take 2 capsules by mouth after meals and at bedtime.

1d   Inject 5 units of insulin subcutaneously now.

1e   Give 1 gram of Ancef® by intravenous piggyback every 6 hours.

1f   Take 10 mg of Inderal® by mouth four times a day.

1g   Take 1 Dalmane® 15-mg capsule by mouth at bedtime.

1h   Take 2 puffs of Atrovent® inhaler 4 times a day as directed.

1i   Instill 2 drops of Cortisporin® otic in both ears three times a day.

1j   Take 1 teaspoonful of Cefzil® twice a day for 10 days.

1k   Take 2 Persantine® 50-mg tablets 4 times a day, 30 minutes before meals.

2   Patient name, drug name, dose, route, dosage regimen, date (and time), and signature

3   1 capsule × 4 doses × 10 days = 40 capsules

4   Change 0.03 g to 30,000 mcg   200 mcg/1 dose =
      30,000 mcg/?   ? = 150 doses

5   2 mg × 3 times a day × 30 days = 180 mg = 0.18 gram

6   4 fl oz = 120 ml = 24 tsp   24 tsp/6 days = ?/1 day
      ? = 4 tsp/day

NOTE: It is OK to work problem 6 and all the remaining problems any way you prefer as long as you understand what you are doing and get the correct answers.
You might have solved this last problem as:
120 ml/6 days = ?/1 day
? = 20 ml per day or 4 teaspoonfuls

NOTE: Beginning with the next question, I will be converting to units in this answer key without further explanation. I believe you are advancing enough to recognize when conversions have been made. In Question 7, there are four different units, i.e., milligrams, grams, fluid ounces, and tablespoons. I converted grams to milligrams because the answer is asked for in milligrams. I converted the fluid ounces to tablespoons because it was just a lot easier for me.
Good luck and hang in there!

7   360 mg/12 tbsp = ?/1 tbsp ? = 30 mg per tablespoonful

8   50 mcg/1 ml = 500 mcg/? ? = 10 ml

9   1 inhal./50 mcg = 200 inhal./? ? = 10,000 mcg = 10 mg

10   5 ml × 3 × 10 = 150 ml

11   200 mcg/1 ml = 125 mcg/? ? = 0.625 ml

12   120 ml/1 day = 960 ml/?   ? = 8 days

13   50 mg/5 ml = ?/120 ml   ? = 1,200 mg

14   50 u/1 ml = ?/20 ml   ? = 1000 u/hr × 24 hours =
      24,000 units per day

15   (10 u × 4 = 40 u/day) (100 u/ml = ?/10 ml   then
      ? = 1000 units per vial)
      40 units/1 day = 1000 units/? ? = 25 days

16   3 mg/2.2 lb = ?/36 lb   ? = 49.1 mg
      (Did you catch my shortcut?)

17   30 mg/5 ml = 49.1 mg/?   ? = 8.183 ml = 8.2 ml

18   (25 mg/2.2 lb = ?/220 lb   ? = 2,500 mg/day × 7 days =
      17,500 mg per week)
      500 mg/1 capsule = 17,500 mg/?   ? = 35 capsules

19   325 mg/1 tablet = ?/42 tablets   ? = 13,650 mg

20	13,650 mg/20 kg = ?/1 kg
	? = 682.5 mg (i.e., 682.5 mg/kg)

21	2 puffs × 6 × 42 days = 504 puffs for the vacation
	200 puffs/1 canister = 504 puffs/?
	? = 2.52 canisters (take **3** on trip)

22	2 mg/1 lb = ?/8.8 lb
	? = 17.6 mg/day × 5 days = 88 mg total

23	10 ml × 3 × 3 days = 90 ml *then* 5 ml × 3 ×
	4 days = 60 ml 60 ml + 90 ml = 150 ml total
	150 ml/30 ml per fl.oz. = 5 fl.oz.

24	0.4 mg alkaloid/15 ml = ?/1000 ml
	? = 26.67 mg of alkaloid

25	$78.50/960 ml = ?/15 ml ? = $1.23

CHAPTER 5

1a	a.a. means "of each"
1b	ad. means "add *up to*"
1c	q.s. means "add a sufficient quantity *to make*"
1d	D.T.D. means "give of such doses"
1e	M. means "mix"
1f	ft. means "make"

2	325 mg aceta./1 tab = ?/5,000 tabs
	? = 1,625,000 mg = 1,625 g

3a	30 mg pseudoephedrine × 100 = 3,000 mg = 3 grams
3b	2 mg brompheniramine × 100 = 200 mg = 0.2 gram
3c	200 mg ibuprofen × 100 = 20,000 mg = 20 grams

4	12.5 mg/5 ml = ?/480 ml ? = 1,200 mg = 1.2 grams

5	500 mg/1 tablet = ?/150 tablets
	? = 75,000 mg or 75 grams per bottle
	75 grams/1 bottle = ?/10,000 bottles
	? = 750,000 g = 750 kg

6a	NOTE: The total formula weight is 10 + 2 + 88 = 100 g.
	10 g pre.sul./100 g = ?/2000 g
	? = 200 g of precipitated sulfur
6b	2 g sal.ac./100 g = ?/2000 g ? = 40 g of salicylic acid
6c	88 g hydr.ung./100 g = ?/2000 g
	? = 1,760 g of hydrophilic oint.

NOTE: The easiest way to answer 6c would be to create a factor 2000/100 = 20 and multiply everything by the 20. To check your answer, *add* all three components together; they should total 2,000 g or 2 kg.

7a	10 g pre.sul./100 g = ?/60 g
	? = 6 g of precipitated sulfur
7b	2 g sal.ac/100 g = ?/60g ? = 1.2 g of salicylic acid
7c	88 g hydr.ung./100 g = ?/60 g
	? = 52.8 g of hydrophilic oint.

NOTE: An easier solution to 7c is to multiply by the factor 0.6, i.e., 60/100. Check your answer by adding all the components together, i.e., 6 + 1.2 + 52.8 = 60 g.

NOTE: Question 8a can be worked by ratio and proportion, but let's take the shortcut and create a factor to multiply times each component. The factor is 45/120 = 0.375.

8a	Camphor = 0.375 × 0.3 g = 0.1125 g camphor
8b	Menthol = 0.375 × 2 g = 0.75 g menthol
8c	Talc = 0.375 × 90 g = 33.75 g talc
8d	Zinc oxide **(If you multiplied 120 × 0.375, you *killed* the patient! Do not forget, *qs* to 120 g means you add up the other components and subtract them from 120 g to find out how much zinc oxide is needed. In this case, 0.3 + 2 + 90 = 92.3 g, then**

120 – 92.3 = 27.7 g of zinc oxide in the original formula. Now multiply this by the factor of 0.375.)
zinc oxide = 0.375 × 27.7 g = 10.39 g zinc oxide
Now add them together to see if you get 45 g as a final answer.   0.1125 + 0.75 + 33.75 + 10.39 = 45 g

9a	0.3 g camphor/120 g = ?/454 g ? = 1.135 g camphor
9b	2 g menthol/120 g = ?/454 g ? = 7.57 g menthol
9c	90 g talc/120 g = ?/454 g ? = 340.5 g talc
9d	27.7 g zinc oxide/120 g = ?/454 g ? = 104.8 g zinc oxide

NOTE: The factor for problem 9d is 454/120 = 3.783, and all four quantities add up to 454 g.

10	90 ml glycerin/1000 ml = ?/480 ml
	? = 43.2 ml glycerin to make a pint

11	70 ml ipecac/1000 ml = ?/3840 ml
	? = 268.8 ml of ipecac fl. extract/gal

12a	75 mcg/1 capsule = ?/30 capsules
	? = 2,250 mcg = 2.2 mg reserpine
12b	20 mg furosemide/1 cap = ?/30 caps
	? = 600 mg = 0.6 g furosemide
12c	15 mg + 0.075 mg + 20 mg = 35.075 mg per capsule
12d	35.075 mg/1 capsule = ?/30 capsules
	? = 1,052.25 mg = 1.052 grams
12e	15 mg hydralazine/30 caps = ?/1 cap
	? = 0.5 mg = 500 mcg hydral./cap

CHAPTER 6

1a	125 mg/5 ml = ?/200 ml ? = 5,000 mg ampicillin in bottle
1b	200 ml final volume – 158 ml of diluent = 42 ml dry powder volume
1c	178 ml diluent + 42 ml powder volume = 220 ml
1d	5000 mg/220 ml = ?/10 ml ? = 227.3 mg ampicillin
1e	5000 mg/220 ml = 250 mg/? ? = 11 ml

2a	125 mg/5 ml = ?/150 ml ? = 3,750 mg cefaclor per bottle
2b	150 ml final volume – 111 ml diluent = 39 ml dry volume
2c	100 mg/5 ml = 3750 mg/? ? = 187.5 ml
	187.5 ml – 150 ml = 37.5 ml of additional water
2d	78 ml diluent + 39 ml dry volume = 117 ml final volume
	3750 mg/117 ml = ?/5 ml ? = 160.3 mg per 5 ml
2e	3750 mg/117 ml = 100 mg/? ? = 3.12 ml

3a	100 mg/1 ml = 300 mg/? ? = 3 ml
3b	100 mg/1 ml = ?/10 ml ? = 1000 mg = 1 gram/vial
3c	250 mg × 4 × 10 days = 10,000 mg total
	1000 mg/1 vial = 10,000 mg/? ? = 10 vials
3d	10 ml final volume – 7.8 ml diluent = 2.2 ml dry volume
3e	9.8 ml diluent + 2.2 ml dry volume = 12 ml final volume
	1000 mg/12 ml = 250 mg/? ? = 3 ml

4a	500,000 u/1 ml = 2,500,000 u/? ? = 5 ml
4b	500,000 u/1 ml = 10,000,000 u/? ? = 20 ml
4c	20 ml final volume – 7 ml powder volume = 13 ml of diluent
4d	20 ml diluent + 7 ml powder volume = 27 ml final volume
	10,000,000 u/27 ml = ?/1 ml ? = 370,370 units/ml
4e	10,000,000 u/27 ml = 2,500,000 u/? ? = 6.75 ml

CHAPTER 7

1a	1200 ml/8 hr = ?/1 hr ? = 150 ml/hr
1b	1200 ml/480 min = ?/5 min ? = 12.5 ml per 5 min
1c	15 gtt/1 ml = ?/1200 ml ? = 18,000 drops
1d	18,000 gtt/480 min = ?/1 min ? = 37.5 gtt/min
1e	2000 mg/8 hr = ?/1 hr ? = 250 mg per hour

NOTE: You probably worked some of these differently and that is cool as long as your answers were correct. I can think of numerous ways to work these problems.

2a 500 ml/480 min = ?/1 min   ? = 1.042 ml per minute
2b 60 gtt/ml = ?/1.042 ml   ? = 62.5 = 63 drops per min
2c 2 ml/1 min = 500 ml/?   ? = 250 minutes
2d 60 gtt/1 ml = ?/2 ml   ? = 120 drops per minute
2e 2000 mcg/500 ml = ?/1 ml   ? = 4 mcg per ml

3a 15 gtt/ml = 40 gtt/?   ? = 2.67 ml per minute
3b 2.67 ml/1 min = ?/1440 min   ? = 3,845 ml per day
3c Looks like 3.845 liters or 4 liter bags
3d 2.67 ml/1 hr = ?/60 min   ? = 160 ml per hour
    1000 mg drug/1000 ml = ?/160 ml   ? = 160 mg per hour
3e 160 mg/60 min = ?/1 min
    ? = 2.67 mg = 2,670 mcg per minute

4a 1000 ml/6 hr = ?/1 hr   ? = 166.7 ml/hr
4b 2,000,000 u/6 hr = ?/1 hr   ? = 333,333 units per hour
4c 2,000,000 u/360 min = ?/1 min
    ? = 5,556 units per minute
4d 1000 ml/360 min = ?/1 min   ? = 2.78 ml per minute
4e 1000 ml/6 hr = ?/1 hr   ? = 166.7 ml/hr
    12 gtt/1 ml = ?/166.7 ml   ? = 2,000 drops per hour
4f 12 gtt/1 ml = ?/1000 ml   ? = 12,000 total drops
    2,000,000 u/12,000 gtt = ?/1 gtt   ? = 166.7 units/drop

5a 100 mg/1 hr = ?/24 hr   ? = 2,400 mg = 2.4 grams
5b 2400 mg/2000 ml = 100 mg/?   ? = 83.3 ml per hour
5c 2000 ml/1440 min = ?/1 min   ? = 1.39 ml per minute
5d 15 gtt/1 ml = ?/1.39 ml
    ? = 20.85 = 21 drops per minute
5e 2000 ml/24 hours = ?/5 hours   ? = 416.7 ml in 5 hours
5f 100 mg/1 hour = ?/3.5 hours   ? = 350 mg in 3½ hours

CHAPTER 8

1a 18.75% 3/16 0.1875 3:16*
    *(incorrectly written, to be discussed later)
1b 18.18%   2/11   0.1818   2:11*
1c 18% 18/100 0.18 18:100* (should be reduced)
1d 3.5% 3.5/100 0.035 3.5:100*
1e 61% 61/100 0.61 61:100*
1f 8% 8/100 0.08 8:100* (should be reduced)
1g 0.8% 1/125 0.008 1:125 (This is the only correctly
    written ratio)
1h 8.75% 35/400 0.0875 35:400* (should be reduced)

2a 12 fl oz/128 fl oz (gallon) = ?/100 fl oz ? = 9.375/100 =
    9.375%
2b 1 pint/8 pints (gallon) = ?/100 pints ? = 12.5/100 =
    12.5%
2c 480 ml + 960 ml + 180 ml + 180 ml + 120 ml = 1920 ml
    (you could also work in ounces)
    1920 ml/3840 ml (gallon) =
    ?/100 ml   ? = 50/100 = 50%
2d 100% − 50% = 50% (left over for the rest of my herd!)

**I will give you all future answers in percent. I assume you
understand that it means ?/100.**

3a 5 trout/30 trout = ?/100 trout   ? = 16.7%
3b 20 trout/30 trout = ?/100 trout   ? = 66.7%
3c 2.2 lb/1 kg = 22.5 lb/?   ? = 10.23 kg
3d 950 g/10,230 g = ?/100 g   ? = 9.29%
3e 18 escaped/48 total (30 + 18) = ?/100 trout
    ? = 37.5% escaped

4   25 g fat/100 g steak = ?/454 g steak
    ? = 113.5 g of fat (yuck!)

5   4 oz fat/14 oz chops = ?/100 oz chops
    ? = 28.6% fat (yuckier!)

6   21 miles/26.2 miles = ?/100 miles   ? = 80.2%

7a 28 g protein/448 g beans = ?/100 g beans
    ? = 6.25% protein

7b 2 g fat/100 g beans = ?/448 g beans   ? = 8.96 g fat
7c 448 g total − 68 g carbohydrate = 380 g are not
    carbohydrate; 380 g non-carbs/448 g beans =
    ?/100 g beans   ? = 84.8% non-carbohydrate

8a 12 g coal tar/150 g ung = ?/100 g ung   ? = 8% coal tar
8b Answer 8% (This is a biggie! If the final product is 8%,
    then 1 g, 1 kg, 1 oz, 1 lb, 1 ton, etc., of the product is
    still 8%. **Please** do not forget this.) To prove my point
    let's check our answer. 12,000 mg C.T./150,000 mg ung
    = ?/100 mg   ? = 8 mg or (8 mg/100 mg = 0.08 = 8%)

9a 2 mg drug/1 g powder = ?/ 120 g powder
    ? = 240 mg drug in 120 g
9b 2 mg drug/1000 mg powder = ?/100 mg powder
    ? = 0.2% drug in powder

10a 3 g hydrocortisone/100 g cream = ?/454 g cream
     ? = 13.62 g hydrocortisone

**NOTE: To check your answer, take the amount of
hydrocortisone and divide it by the total weight of the
product.   Check   13.62/454 = 0.03 = 3%**

10b 3 g hydrocortisone/100 g cream = ?/1 g cream
     ? = 0.03 g = 30 mg

11a 5 g fluorouracil/100 g cream = ?/25 g cream
     ? = 1.25 g = 1,250 mg
11b 5% means you have 1.25 g in the 25 g of cream. If you
     add 2 more g of fluorouracil, you will now have 3.25 g of
     fluorouracil (1.25 + 2 = 3.25), but you must also
     remember to increase the final or total weight of the
     cream by 2 grams, giving a final weight of 27 g
     (25 + 2 = 27). Now solve the question.
     3.25 g fluorouracil/27 g cream = ?/100 g cream
     ? = 12.04%

12a 1.5 g hydrocortisone/60 g cream = ?/100 g cream
     ? = 2.5%
12b 60 g total − 2 g hydro and Vio® (i.e., 1.5 + 0.5 = 2)
     = 58 grams of cream base
12c 1 oz (weight)/28.4 grams = 10 oz/?
     ? = 284 grams of product
     0.5 g Vioform/60 g product = ?/284 g product
     ? = 2.37 g Vioform powder

13a 200 mg aminophylline/1 sup. = ?/60 sup.
     ? = 12,000 mg = 12 g
13b 60 mg + 200 mg + 1,800 mg = 2,060 mg
     (weight of 1 suppository) = 2.06 grams
     2.06 g/1 suppos. = ?/60 suppos.   ? = 123.6 grams
13c As mentioned in Question 8b, whatever the percent is for
     1 suppository, it will be the same for 60 suppositories.
     The total weight for 1 suppository is 2,060 mg.
     60 mg phen/2060 mg total wgt. = ?/100 mg wgt.
     ? = 2.91% phenobarbital

14a 1 g benzocaine/1000 g product = ?/120 g product
     ? = 0.12 g = 120 mg
14b 10 g pre.sul/100 g product = ?/1000 g product
     ? = 100 g precipitated sulfur
     (Check: 100 g sulfur/1000 g product = 0.1 = 10%)

15a Total parts = 14 (2 + 5 + 7 = 14) Now you decide what
     a part is. I picked grams. 7 g Ca.carb/14 g powder =
     ?/908 g powder (2 lb)   ? = 454 g calcium carb.
15b 5 parts/14 parts = ?/100 parts
     ? = 35.7% sodium bicarb.
15c 2 parts magnesium oxide to 14 total parts →
     2:14 reduced to 1:7

16a 0.35 ml mint/100 ml m-wash = ?/960 ml m-wash
     ? = 3.36 ml mint flavoring
16b I hope you did not miss this! It is still 0.35% mint flavoring.

17a 16 ml resorcinol/180 ml lotion = ?/100 ml lotion
     ? = 8.89% resorcinol
17b 16 ml resorcinol/180 ml lotion = ?/5000 ml lotion
     ? = 444.4 ml resorcinol

18a 6 ml menthyl/100 ml lotion = 480 menthyl/?
     ? = 8000 ml = 2.083 gal.
18b 6 ml menthyl/100 ml lotion = ?/480 ml lotion
     ? = 28.8 ml menthyl sal.
     Check: 28.8 ml menthyl sal./480 ml lotion = 0.06 = 6%

19   5 ml oil/100 ml *spirits* = 15 ml oil/?
     ? = 300 ml *spirits*

20   1 ml oil/15 ml *spirits* = 240 ml oil/?
     ? = 3,600 ml *spirits*

21a 0.9 g Sod.Cl/100 ml sol. = ?/1000 ml sol.
     ? = 9 g sodium chloride
21b 200 ml/1 hr = ?/3 hr   ? = 600 ml
     0.9 g NaCl/100 ml = ?/600 ml   ? = 5.4 grams NaCl

22a 37.5 g Na Bicarb/500 ml = ?/100 ml
     ? = 7.5% sodium bicarb.
22b 37.5 g Na Bicarb/500 ml = ?/100 ml
     ? = 7.5 g = 7500 mg Na Bicarb

NOTE: You could also use your answer from 22a and say 100 ml × 7.5% = 7.5 g.

22c Please tell me you got this right this time!
     It is 7.5% no matter what the volume.

23a 85 g iodine/3840 ml = ?/100 ml   ? = 2.21%
23b 3 g iodine/100 ml tincture = 85 g iodine/?
     ? = 2,833 ml 3% tincture
23c 1 g iodine/100 ml tincture = 85 g iodine/?
     ? = 8,500 ml 1:100 tincture

24a 25 mg adenosine/1 ml = ?/10 ml
     ? = 250 mg = 0.25 gram
24b 25 mg/1 ml = ?/100 ml   ? = 2500 mg/100 ml =
     2.5 g/100 ml = 2.5%
24c 25 mg adenosine/1 ml = 35 mg adenosine/?   ? = 1.4 ml

25a 0.5 g pilocarpine/100 ml sol. = ?/15 ml
     ? = 0.075 g = 75 mg
25b 18 drops/1 ml = ?/15 ml   ? = 270 drops per bottle
25c 75 mg/270 drops = ?/1 drop
     ? = 0.278 mg = 278 mcg/gtt

26a 50 mg nitro/1000 ml = ?/100 ml   ? = 5 mg/100 ml =
     0.005 g/100 ml = 0.005%
26b 50,000 mcg nitro/1000 ml = 200 mcg nitro/?
     ? = 4 ml solution

27   5 g drug/100 ml = 0.015 g (test dose)/?
     ? = 0.3 ml of the 5% sol.

28   200 mg/dL → 200 mg/100 ml → 0.2 g/100 ml → 0.2%

29   0.15% → 0.15 g/100 ml → 150 mg/100 ml →150 mg%
     or (150 mg/dL)

30   95 mg% → 95 mg/100 ml
     95 mg cholesterol/100 ml = ?/1 ml
     ? = 0.95 mg = 950 mcg

31a 8 ppm → 8/1,000,000 → 1/125,000 → 1:125,000
31b 8/1,000,000 = 0.000008 = 0.0008%
31c 8 g antifungal/1,000,000 g feed = ?/1000 g feed
     ? = 0.008 g antifungal

32   1 g sod.fluoride/1,000,000 ml = ?/3,840,000 ml
     ? = 3.84 g sodium fluoride

33   0.00005 g/100 ml = ?/1,000,000 ml
     ? = 0.5 g/1,000,000 = 0.5 ppm

34   0.00005 g/100 ml = ?/1000 ml
     ? = 0.0005 g = 500 mcg

35a 2/7 = 1/?   ? = 3.5   2:7 → 1:3.5
35b 17/510 = 1/?   ? = 30   17:510 → 1:30
35c 33/135 = 1/?   ? = 4.1   33:135 → 1:4.1
35d 0.125 → 125/1000 → 125:1000 → 1:8
     (I just reduced this one, but you can work it either way.)
35e 0.08 → 8/100 → 8:100 → 8/100 = 1/?   ? = 12.5
     8:100 → 1:12.5
35f 0.45 → 45/100 = 1/?   ? = 2.22 45:100 → 1:2.22
35g 2:23 → 2/23 = 1/?   ? = 11.5 2:23 →   1:11.5
35h 23:300 → 23/300 = 1/?   ? = 13.04 23:300 → 1:13.04
35i 48:200 → 48/200 = 1/?   ? = 4.167 48:200 → 1:4.167

NOTE: To check your answers, divide the ratios and see if the *decimal fractions* are similar. *Example* (35i) above: 48/200 = 0.24   and   1/4.167 = 0.24

CHAPTER 9

1
     12 techs × 100 Rx = 1200 techsRx
     20 techs × 125 Rx = 2500 techsRx
     23 techs × 150 Rx = 3450 techsRx
      8 techs × 175 Rx = 1400 techsRx
     ──────────   ──────────
     63 techs   8550 techsRx

     8550 techsRx/**63** techs = **135.7 Rx (per tech)**
     ("techs" cancel out.)

2
     2 liters   × 20% = 40 liter %
     1 liter   × 50% = 50 liter %
     0.75 liter × 80% = 60 liter %
     ──────────   ──────────
     3.75 liters   **150** liter%

     (Make sure all units are the same. I selected liters, but mls are OK.)
     150 liter%/**3.75** liters = **40%**

NOTE: I frequently see mistakes with this type of problem when students accidentally add the middle column or divide by the wrong numbers. Please be careful.

(Of course you would not make a mistake like that because you always ESTIMATE the correct answer. Right?)

3
     1 pint   ×   10% = 10 pint%
     6 pints ×   5% = 30 pint%
     8 pints ×   20% = 160 pint%
     ──────────   ──────────
     15 pints   **200** pint %

     200 pint%/**15** pints = **13.33%**

4
     15 pints × 13.33% = 200 pint%
      2 pints ×   0% =   0 pint%
     ──────────   ──────────
     17 pints   **200** pint%

     200 pint%/**17** pints = **11.76%**

5
     480 ml   × 2% =   960 ml%
     1000 ml × 6% = 6000 ml%
     ──────────   ──────────
     1480 ml   **6960** ml%

     6960 ml%/**1480** ml = **4.7%**

6
     1480 ml × 4.7% = 6956 ml%
      500 ml × 0.2% =   100 ml%
     ──────────   ──────────
     1980 ml   **7056** ml%

     7056 ml%/**1980** ml = **3.56%**

7
1000 ml × 95% = 95000 ml%
960 ml × 70% = 67200 ml%
480 ml × 0% = 0 ml%
2440 ml   162,200 ml%
(480 ml is 17% benzalkonium chloride **BUT** 0% alcohol.)
162,200 ml%/2440 ml = 66.48%

8
5% + 15% + 20 % = 40%   40%/3 = **13.33%**
(This is like your English test average, but a lot lower. You can also work this by alligation medial if you wish.)

9
300 grams × 13.33% = 4000 gram%
100 grams × 100% = 10000 gram%
400 grams   **14000** gram%

14000 gram%/**400** grams = **35%**

10
454 grams × 2% = 908 gram%
1000 grams × 5% = 5000 gram%
1454 grams   **5908** gram%

5908 gram%/**1454** grams = **4.06%**

11a
(OV) (O%) = (NV) (N%)
(30 ml) (10%) = (1000 ml) (N%)   0.3% = N%
11b   0.3% = 0.3/100   0.3/100 = 1/?   ? = 333 → 1:333
11c   0.3 g/100 ml = ?/15 ml   ? = 0.045 gram tablespoonful
11d   10 g/100 ml = ?/5 ml   ? = 0.5 gram/teaspoonful

12a
(OV) (O%) = (NV) (N%)
(120) (10%) = (NV) (1%)   1200 ml = NV
12b   1200 ml – 120 ml = 1080 ml
of diluent to be added to the 120 ml of 10% stock.

13
(OV) (O%) = (NV) (N%)
(OV) (17%) = (1000) (0.5%)   OV = 29.4 ml

14
0.5 g/100 ml = ?/30 ml   ? = 0.15 gram = 150 mg

15
(OV) (O%) = (NV) (N%)
(10) (O%) = (1000) (0.5%)   O% = 50%

16
50 g/100 ml = ?/480 ml   ? = 240 grams in the 50% stock bottle

17a
(OV) (O%) = (NV) (N%)
(1 oz) (5%) = (5 oz) (N%)   1% = N%

NOTE: We **added** 4 oz to the 1 oz of 5% = 5 oz total.

17b   1% = 1/100 = 1:100

18
(OV) (O%) = (NV) (N%)
(OV) (2%) = (960) (0.05%)   OV = 24 ml

19
(OV) (O%) = (NV) (N%)
(480) (95%) = (NV) (20%)   2280 ml = NV

NOTE: This is the _final_ dilution, but it is not the answer to the question. If we started with a pint and finished with 2280 ml, then we had to add a diluent to the pint to get 2280 ml. The correct volume that was _added_ is 2280 – 480 = 1800 ml.

20a
(OV) (O%) = (NV) (N%)
(100) (50%) = (500) (N%)   10% = N%

NOTE: Again, 400 ml was _added_ to 100 ml to make a final volume of 500 ml. Be very careful in reading these dilution questions.

20b
(OV) (O%) = (NV) (N%)
(100) (50%) = (NV) (5%)   1000 ml = NV
20c   1000 ml – 100 ml = 900 ml to be added

20d
(OV) (O%) = (NV) (N%)
(100) (50%) = (1100) (N%)
NOTE: 100 ml of 50% + 1000 ml of **0% dextrose**. It is 0.9% NaCl, but 0% dextrose. 4.55% = N%

21
GOTCHA! You cannot add a 6% and 50% ointment and have a 4%. As mentioned earlier, your answer has to be between the 6% and 50% ointments.

22a

```
95%          10 parts
      55%
45%          40 parts
```

Answer: 10 parts of 95% added to 40 parts of the 45%
22b   Total parts equal 50 parts of the 55% final product (i.e., 10 + 40 = 50)   50 parts/1000 ml = 10 parts/?
? = 200 ml of the 95% alcohol
22c   50 parts/1000 ml = 40 parts/?
? = 800 ml of the 45% alcohol

NOTE: The shortcut is: 1000 ml final product – 200 ml of 95% = 800 ml.

22d
This question is limited by the quantity in least supply; in this case, 1 pint of 95%.
10 parts/480 ml = 50 parts/?
? = 2,400 ml of 55% can be made.

23a

```
100%         3 parts
      5%
2%           95 parts
```

23b _Answer:_ 3 parts of 100% added to 95 parts of 2%
98 parts/454 g = 95 parts/?
? = 440.1 g of the 2% needed
23c   454 – 440.1 = 13.9 grams of the 100% coal tar needed. (Can also be done with ratios.)
23d   3 parts/113.5 grams = 98 parts/?
? = 3707.7 grams = 3.708 kg

24a

```
20%          2 parts
      12%
10%          8 parts
```

24b _Answer:_ 2 parts of 20% mixed with 8 parts of 10%
10 parts/480 ml = 8 parts/?
? = 384 ml of the 10% solution.
24c   12 grams/100 ml = ?/480 ml
? = 57.6 grams KCl/pint of 12%
24d   12 grams/100 ml = ?/15 ml
? = 1.8 grams = 1,800 milligrams
24e   You can work this by alligation, but, since you are using a **zero percent diluent**, you can work this as a simple dilution: (OV) (O%) = (NV) (N%)
(OV) (20%) = (1000) (12%)
OV = 600 ml of the 20%
Answer: 1000 – 600 = **400 ml** diluent

25a
YES, you can mix a 20% with a 1% and make an intermediate strength of 2%.
25b   1 part × 20% = 20 part%
1 part × 1% = 1 part%
2 parts   21 part%
21 part%/2 parts = 10.5% lidocaine
25c   30 ml × 1% = 30 ml%
20 ml × 20% = 400 ml%
50 ml   430 ml%
430 ml%/50 ml = 8.6% lidocaine
25d   0.4 g/100 ml = ?/1 ml
? = 0.004 g = 4 milligrams
25e   30 ml/1 hr = ?/24 hr
? = 720 ml of 5% dextrose in 24 hours
5 grams/100 ml = ?/720 ml
? = 36 grams of dextrose/day

CHAPTER 10

1a 10 g KCl/100 ml = ?/480 ml   ? = 48 grams KCl/pint

1b MW KCl = 74.5   valence = 1   then   74.5 mg/1 = 74.5 mg per mEq   74.5 mg/1 mEq = 48,000 mg/?
? = 644.3 mEq KCl/pint

1c 644.3 mEq potassium (see "statement of unity" discussion)

1d 644.3 mEq KCl/480 ml = ?/15 ml
? = 20.1 mEq KCl/tablespoon

1e 10 mEq q.i.d. = 40 mEq daily
644.3 mEq/480 ml = 40 mEq/?
? = 29.8 ml = 30 ml

2a MW NaCl = 58.5   valence = 1   then   58.5 mg/1 = 58.5 mg per mEq   58.5 mg/1 mEq = 1000 mg/?
? = 17.1 mEq NaCl per tablet

2b 1 tab × 3 × 7 days = 21 tablets
1 tablet/17.1 mEq = 21 tablets/?
? = 359 mEq NaCl → 359 mEq Na

2c 17.1 mEq Na/1 tab = 100 mEq Na/?
? = 5.84 tablets = 6 tablets

3 1 mEq NaCl/58.5 mg = 154 mEq NaCl/?
? = 9009 mg = 9.009 grams NaCl

4 9.009 g/1000 ml = ?/100 ml
? = 0.9 g/100 ml = 0.9% (normal saline)

5a 1 mEq NaCl = 58.5 mg   1 mEq Na/1 kg = ?/72 kg
? = 72 mEq   1 mEq NaCl/58.5 mg = 72 mEq NaCl/?
? = 4,212 mg NaCl

5b 1 mEq/2.2 lb = ?/110 lb   ? = 50 mEq NaCl
1 mEq NaCl/58.5 mg = 50 mEq/?
? = 2,925 mg = 2.925 grams

5c 0.9 g NaCl/100 ml = 2.925 g NaCl/?
? = 325 ml of NS

5d 14.6 g NaCl/100 ml = 2.925 g NaCl/?
? = 20 ml of 14.6% NaCl

6 100 ml/1 hr = ?/24 hr   ? = 2,400 ml daily
0.9 g NaCl/100 ml = ?/2400 ml   ? = 21.6 g NaCl daily
58.5 mg NaCl/1 mEq = 21600 mg NaCl/?
? = 369 mEq Na daily

7a MW CaCl$_2$ = 111   valence = 2
then 111 mg/2 = 55.5 mg per mEq
1 mEq CaCl$_2$/55.5 mg = 30 mEq CaCl$_2$/?
? = 1,665 mg calcium chloride

7b 1.665 grams/1000 ml = ?/100 ml
? = 0.1665% calcium chloride

8a MW NaHCO$_3$ = 84   valence = 1   then
84 mg/1 = 84 mg per mEq
90 mEq/100 ml = ?/1000 ml
? = 900 mEq   1 mEq/84 mg = 900 mEq/?
? = 75,600 mg per liter

8b 75.6 grams/1000 ml = ?/100 ml   ? = 7.56%

9a MW NH$_4$Cl = 53.5   valence = 1 then 53.5 mg/1 = 53.5 mg per mEq   1 mEq/53.5 mg = 100 mEq/?
? = 5350 mg = 5.35 g   5.35 g/20 ml = ?/100 ml
? = 26.75% ammonium chloride

9b 5.35 g/520 ml = ?/100 ml   ? = 1.03%
(500 + 20 = 520 ml)

10a MW NaC$_2$H$_3$O$_2$ = 82   valence = 1
then 82 mg/1 = 82 mg per mEq
1 mEq/82 mg = 4 mEq/?   ? = 328 mg per ml
328 mg/1 ml = 1000 mg/?   ? = 3.05 ml

10b 4 mEq/1 ml = ?/5 ml   ? = 20 mEq of sodium acetate = 20 mEq sodium (see "statement of unity")

10c 0.328 g/1 ml = ?/100 ml   ? = 32.8%

CHAPTER 11

1a °C = (°F − 32) ÷ 1.8   (Use this formula for 1a–1e.)
= (41 − 32) ÷ 1.8
= 9 ÷ 1.8 = **5 °C**

1b = (86 − 32) ÷ 1.8 = 54 ÷ 1.8 = **30°C**

1c = (167 − 32) ÷ 1.8 = 135 ÷ 1.8 = **75°C**

1d = (14 − 32) ÷ 1.8 = (−18) ÷ 1.8 = **−10 °C**

1e = (− 40 − 32) ÷ 1.8 = (−72) ÷ 1.8 = **−40°C**
(same value)

2a °F = (1.8 × °C) + 32 (Use this formula for 2a–2e.)
= (1.8 × 15) + 32
= (27) + 32 = **59°F**

2b = (1.8 × 75) + 32 = 135 + 32 = **167°F**

2c = (1.8 × 0) + 32 = 0 + 32 = **32°F**

2d = (1.8 × −5) + 32 = −9 + 32 = **23°F**

2e = (1.8 × −75) + 32 = −135 + 32 = **−103°F**

CHAPTER 12

1a $78 − $45 = $33 markup

1b $78 − $45/$78 = 33/78 = 0.42 = 42%
markup based on selling price

1c $78 − $45/$45 = 33/45 = 0.73 = 73%
markup based on cost

1d 1.72 × $45 = $77.40
(selling price based on 72% markup on cost)

1e 100% − 72% = 28% (cost of the product)
28%/100% = $45/?   ? = $160.71
(selling price based on 72% markup based on selling price)

2a $78 − $12 = $66

2b $78/60 tablets = ?/1 tablet   ? = $1.30 per tablet

2c $12/60 tablets = ?/1 tablet   ? = $0.20

2d 1 tab × 2 × 7 days = 14 tablets/wk
60 tablets/$78 = 14 tablets/?   ? = $18.20

2e 78 − 66/66 = 12/66 = 0.182 = 18.2% markup
based on cost.

2f 78 − 66/78 = 12/78 = 0.154 = 15.4% markup
based on selling price

3a G.P. = sales − cost = $4,300,000 − $2,670,000 = $1,630,000

3b NP = GP − overhead = $1,630,000 − $850,000 = $780,000

3c 100%/$780,000 = 5%/?   ? = $39,000
(If you don't want it, I'll take it!)

3d Inventory turnover rate = total purchases/average inventory ITR = $2,670,000/$520,000 = 5.13 times

3e $62/1 sale = $4,300,000/?   ? = 69,355 total sales

4a $81,435 − $69,887 = $11,548 monthly gross profit

4b Think about this. If the gross profit is $11,548 and the net profit is $5,328, then the overhead is the difference in these two numbers. Remember the net profit is gross profit minus overhead.
$11,548 − $5,328 = $6,220 overhead

5a 1.20 × $331 = $397.20
(the amount 100 tablets would cost with markup)
100 tablets/$397.20 = 30 tablets/?   ? = $119.16

NOTE: You could also take the cost of 30 tablets ($99.30) and multiply times 1.2 and get the same answer.

5b **100%** total cost after markup − **10%** markup = **90%** original cost of the drug
90% **(cost)** /$331 = 100%   **(selling price)**/?
? = $367.78
NOTE: To check your answer, subtract 10% of the selling price from the selling price and your answer (hopefully) will be the original cost. ($367.78 − $36.78 = $331)

5c $331 × 0.92 = $304.52   or
100%/$331 = 92%/?   ? = $304.52

POSTTEST

NOTE: I will try to trick you on *conversions* throughout this "posttest" so be real careful.

1.   100 capsules/1.44 g = 1 capsule/?
      ? = 0.0144 g = 14.4 milligrams

2.   Total weight = 1.44 + 14.8 + 0.920 + 0.920 + 0.920 +
      30 + 1 = 50 g
      1.44 g neomycin/50 g total = ?/100 g total
      ? = 2.88%

3.   30 g kaolin/100 caps = ?/30 caps
      ? = 9 g = 9,000 milligrams

4.   110 mcg flut./1 actuation = ?/120 acts
      ? = 13,200 mcg = 13.2 milligrams

5.   13.2 mg flut/13,000 mg = ?/100 mg   ? = 0.102%

NOTE: The weight of the contents of the canister is 13 g = 13,000 mg, so it obviously contains more components than the 13.2 mg of fluticasone. The majority of the weight is propellants, preservatives, etc.

6.   20 ml × 2 × 14 = 560 milliliters

7.   Kim receives 40 ml daily
      240 mg drugs/5 ml = ?/40 ml
      ? = 1920 mg = 1.92 grams

8.   0.4 mg/1 hr = ?/12 hr
      ? = 4.8 mg = 4,800 micrograms

9.   1 system/125 mg = 30 systems/?
      ? = 3750 mg = 3.75 grams

10.   240 mg morphine/24 troches = ?/1 troche
      ? = 10 mg morphine per troche

11.   240 mg/24 grams = ?/100 g
      ? = 1000 mg/100 g = 1000 mg%

12.   250 mg NutraSweet®/24 troches = ?/100 troches
      ? = 1042 mg = 1.042 grams

13.   3 tubes × 30 g = 90 grams total of cream in 3 tubes
      0.05 g fluocinonide/100 g cream = ?/90 g cream
      ? = 0.045 g = 45 mg

14.   (OV) (O%) = (NV) (N%)
      (30 g) (0.05%) = (90 g) (N%)   N% = 0.017%

NOTE: This can also be worked by both alligation alternate and alligation medial.

15.   °C = (°F − 32) ÷ 1.8 = (104 − 32) ÷ 1.8 =
      72 ÷ 1.8 = 40°C

16.   50 g/100 ml = ?/2 ml   ? = 1 g per 2-ml vial
      1 g/vial = 20 g/?   ? = 20 vials to provide 20 grams

17.   20 g/500 ml = 4 g/?   ? = 100 ml per hour
      100 ml/60 minutes = ?/1 minute   ? = 1.67 ml/minute

18.   20 gtt/1 ml = ?/1.67 ml
      ? = 33.4 gtt/minute = 33 gtt/min

19.   100 ml/1 hr = ?/24 hr   ? = 2,400 ml in 24 hours
      500 ml/1 bag = 2400 ml/?   ? = 4.8 bags = 5 bags

20.   If *according to directions:* 1 ml contains 100 mg, then
      5 ml must provide the 500 mg listed on the bottle.
      5 ml (final volume) − 4.8 ml (diluent) =
      0.2 ml "dry powder volume"

21.   1 ml/350 mg ceftriaxone = ?/200 mg
      ? = 0.57 milliliter

22.   5 capsules/5 tubes = ?/10 tubes   ? = 10 capsules
      1 capsule/200 mg = 10 capsules/?
      ? = 2000 mg = 2 grams

23.   150 mg/5 tubes = ?/1 tube ? = 30 mg = 0.03 gram

24.   5 tubes × 5 g/tube = 25 grams
      120 mg silica/25 grams = ?/1 gram
      ? = 4.8 mg per gram of formula

25.   430 mg/2 = 215 mg per milliequivalent
      10 g/100 ml = ?/10 ml(vial) ? = 1 gram/vial = 1000 mg
      215 mg/1 mEq = 1000 mg/? ? = 4.65 mEq Ca.gluc./vial

26.   1000 mg/1 vial = ?/25 vials
      ? = 25,000 mg per 25 vials

27.   42 mcg/1 inhalation = 840 mcg/?
      ? = 20 inhalations

28.   42 mcg/1 inhalation = ?/200 inhalations
      ? = 8400 mcg = 8.4 mg per canister
      8.4 mg drug/16.8 g canister = ?/100 g
      ? = 50 mg/100 g = 50 mg%

29.   (OV) (O%) = (NV) (N%)
      (35 ml)(95%) = (100 ml)(N%)
      N% = 33.25% alcohol

30.   5 g progesterone/100 ml = 5%
      NOTE: All volumes of this product will be 5%.

31.   3 g/100 ml = ?/120 ml   ? = 3.6 grams

32.   5 mg Dilantin®/2.2 lb = ?/66 lb
      ? = 150 mg per day ÷ 3 doses = 50 mg/dose
      125 mg/5 ml = 50 mg/?   ? = 2 ml per dose

33.   2 ml × 3 doses = 6 ml per day 6 ml/1 day = 240 ml/?
      ? = 40 days

34.   (OV) (O%) = (NV) (N%)
      (20 ml)(10%) = (100 ml)(N%)
      N% = 2% cyclosporine
      NOTE: 20 + 80 = 100 ml
      NOTE: This can also be worked by alligations. Consider corn oil/olive oil to be 0% cyclosporine.

35.   20 ml cyclo./100 ml sol = ?/60 ml   ? = 12 ml

36.   2 g/100 ml (formulation) = ?/1 ml (formulation)
      ? = 0.02 g = 20 milligrams

37.   2 inhalations 3 times a day = 6 inhalations per day
      6 inhalations/1 day = ?/14 days
      ? = 84 inhalations

38. $68.85/240 inhalations = ?/84 inhalations
      ? = $24.10

39.   °F = (1.8 × °C) + 32
      (1.8 × 20) + 32 = (36) + 32 = 68°F
      (1.8 × 25) + 32 = (45) + 32 = 77°F
      Answer: The range is 68 to 77°F

40.   48 mg sodium per gram Kefzol® and the patient receives
      3 grams daily. 48 × 3 = 144 mg of sodium daily or
      432 mg in 3 days MW sodium = 23 valence = 1 then
      23 mg/1 = 23 mg per mEq
      23 mg/1 mEq = 432 mg/? ? = 18.78 mEq sodium daily

41　8.5 g amino acid/100 ml = 70 g amino acid/?
　　? = 824 ml of 8.5% amino acid sol.

42　420 g dextrose/600 ml = ?/100 ml
　　? = 70% dextrose solution

43　430 mg/2 = 215 mg per mEq
　　215 mg/1 mEq = ?/7 mEq
　　? = 1,505 mg of calcium gluconate

44　1 g/10 ml = 1.505 g/?　? = 15.05 ml = 15 ml

45　3 g testos/100 g gel = ?/454 g gel
　　? = 13.62 grams testosterone

46　(OV) (O%) = (NV) (N%)
　　(87 g) (2%) = (100 g) (N%)　N% = 1.74%

47　10 g/0.84 = 11.9 ml of mineral oil (sp gr 0.84)

48　1 dose/0.25 mg tartaric = 3 doses/?
　　? = 0.75 mg = 750 micrograms

49　58.5 mg/1 = 58.5 mg NaCl per mEq
　　3 mg NaCl/1 ampul = ?/20 ampuls　? = 60 mg NaCl
　　58.5 mg/1 mEq = 60 mg NaCl/?　? = 1.03 mEq NaCl

50　40 g zinc oxide/100 g ung = ?/454,000 g
　　? = 181,600 g = 181.6 kg zinc oxide

51　$1.50 – $1.04/$1.04 = $0.46/$1.04 = 0.442 = 44.2%

52　(OV) (O%) = (NV) (N%)
　　(20 ml) (70%) = (300 ml) (N%)　N% = 4.67%

53　5 ml ban.flav/300 ml = ?/100 ml
　　? = 1.67% banana flavoring

54　2,500,000 units/10 pops = ?/2.5 pops
　　? = 625,000 units nystatin

55　100 ml – 90 ml = 10 ml "dry volume displacement"

56　100 ml water + 10 ml = 110 ml total volume
　　If the 100-ml bottle contains 125 mg Augmentin® per
　　5 ml, then the bottle has a total of 2,500 mg of drug;
　　this does not change as more diluent is added.
　　2,500 mg/110 ml = 125 mg/?
　　? = 5.5-ml dose provides 125 mg

57　Abby is receiving 250 mg per day
　　(125 mg × 2 doses = 250 mg)
　　30 mg/2.2 lb = 250 mg/?　? = 18.33 pounds

58　500 mcg/1 ampule = 250 mcg/?　? = 0.5 ampule, but
　　you will have to send 1 amp. per dose and half of the
　　amp. will be discarded.　Answer 4 amps

59　30 mcg/2.2 lb = ?/14 lb　? = 191 mcg dose
　　250 mcg/1 ml = 191 mcg/?　? = 0.76 ml

60　74.5 mg/1 = 74.5 mg per mEq KCl
　　74.5 mg KCl/1 mEq = 467 mg KCl/?
　　? = 6.27 mEq KCl

61　(OV) (O%) = (NV) (N%)
　　(50 ml) (5%) = (100 ml)(N%)　N% = 25% dextrose

62　95 mg/2 = 47.5 mg/mEq　47.5 mg/1 mEq = 133 mg/?
　　? = 2.8 mEq magnesium chloride

63　75 units/2.2 lb = 5000 units/?　? = 146.7 pounds

64　25,000 units/500 ml = 800 units/?
　　? = 16 milliliters per hour

65　15 gtt/1 ml = ?/16 ml　　　　? = 240 gtt/hr
　　240 gtt/60 minutes = ?/1 minute　? = 4 gtt/minute

66　0.042 g beclomethasone/100 g = ?/25 g
　　? = 0.0105 g = 10.5 milligrams

67　10.5 mg/200 sprays = ?/2 sprays
　　? = 0.105 mg = 105 micrograms

68　100 g total – 54.5 g of other components =
　　45.5 grams of white petrolatum

69　1.5 g cocaine : 100 g total → 1.5/100 = 1/?
　　? = 66.7　　Answer: 1:66.7

70　8 oz = 8 × 28.4 g = 227.2 g
　　3 g phenol/100 g formulation = ?/227.2 g
　　? = 6.82 g phenol crystals

71　1 mg per 1 ml → 100 mg:100 ml →
　　0.1 g:100 ml →
　　1 g:1000 ml → 1:1000

72　0.5 g chloro/100 ml = ?/30 ml
　　? = 0.15 g = 150 mg

73　$1.93 – $0.79/$1.93 = $1.14/$1.93 = 59.1%

74　5000 units/1 g ung = ?/28.4 g
　　? = 142,000 units

75　0.1 mg/2.2 lb = ?/220 lb　? = 10 mg/day divided in
　　2 doses = 5 mg per dose

76　There are 5 mg/ampule which represents a single dose.
　　2 amps/day × 7 days = 14 ampules per week

77　5 ml × 1.04 = 5.2 grams

78　Same as it is for 1 ml of the formula!
　　1.75 g/100 ml = 1.75%

79　1 g piroxicam/100 ml = ?/3840 ml
　　? = 38.4 g piroxicam/gal

80　1:40 dilution is equal to 1/40 is equal to 2.5%

81　2 packets × 4 × 5 days = 40 packets

82　(2 × 2 × 2 = 8 tabs) + (1 × 2 × 3 = 6 tabs)
　　+ (1 × 3 = 3 tabs) = **17 tabs**

83　1 tablet/0.75 mg = 17 tablets/?
　　? = 12.75 mg = 0.01275 g

84　3 g/100 ml = ?/148 ml　　　? = 4.44 grams

85　3 g/100 ml = ?/20,000,000 ml　? = 600,000 g = 600 kg

86　0.1 gram/100 ml = 0.1% idoxuridine

87　2 mg/100 ml = 2 mg%

88　100 mg/100 ml = ?/15 ml
　　? = 15 mg = 15,000 mcg

89　2 inhalations × 2 × 92 days = 368 inhalations
　　100 inhalations/1 canister = 368 inhalations/?
　　? = 3.68 = 4 canisters

90　250 mcg/inhalation = ?/368 inhalations
　　? = 92,000 mcg = 92 mg

91　125 mg/2 ml = 80 mg/?　　　? = 1.28 ml

92   If there are 5 mg/1 ml in a 2-ml amp, then the amp
      contains 10 mg Reglan®. The maximum dose is
      20 mg q6h, which is 80 mg/day.
      10 mg/amp = 80 mg /?   ? = 8 amps

93   The max on the Tylenol® is 2 tablets × 6 doses
      (i.e., q4h) = 12 tablets   1 tablet/325 mg = 12 tablets/?
      ? = 3900 mg = 3.9 grams

94   3.375 g/20 ml = 3 g/?   ? = 17.8 ml

95   If 1 ml (0.2 mg) is diluted to 10 ml, it will contain
      0.02 mg/ml, so the range will be according to
      instructions: 1 ml to 3 ml, which would be
      0.02 mg to 0.06 mg.

96   If you dilute 2 mg in 500 ml, this is the same as
      2,000 mcg per 500 ml. The directions say to give 5 mcg
      per minute. 2000 mcg/500 ml = 5 mcg/?
      ? = 1.25 ml per minute

**NOTE: Theoretically you could consider the final volume
to be 510 ml because the directions for preparation of the
dilution say "dilute 10 ml in 500 ml," but people
routinely ignore small volumes when adding solutions.**

97   1 g/5000 ml = 0.0002 g/?   ? = 1 ml

98   25 g propylene glycol to 100 g total weight →
      25:100 → 1:4

99   13 g sodium stearate/100 g formula = ?/2,750 g
      ? = 357.5 g

100   Alligation alternate should be used since we are adding
      2 different strengths of the *same* drug to make an
      intermediate strength.

      2.5   0.25
          \   /   1.25 parts/28.35 g = 0.25 parts/?
          1.25%   ? = 5.67 g of 2.5%
          /   \
      1   1.25

101   These are different drugs, so the hydrocortisone is
      treated as **0%** desoximetasone. Did I catch you on this
      one? This can be worked by (OV) (O%) = (NV) (N%)
      and by alligation medial. Let's do both solutions
      since this is our last problem.

      (OV) (O%)   = (NV) (N%)
      (15 g) (0.25%) = (43.35 g)(N%) N% = **0.0865%**

      Alligation Medial
      15 grams   × 0.25% = 3.75 grams%
      28.35 grams   ×   0% =   0 grams%
      43.35 grams   3.75 grams%

      3.75 grams%/43.35 grams = 0.0865%

GOOD LUCK!

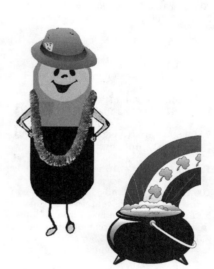